Food Chemical Sensitivity

D1553351

To James.
The purest gold always emerges from the hottest fire.

FOOD CHEMICAL SENSITIVITY

What it is and how to cope with it

Robert Buist PhD

AVERY PUBLISHING GROUP INC.
Garden City Park, New York

First published in 1986 by Harper & Row (Australasia) Pty Ltd.

Copyright © 1988 by Robert Buist

ISBN 0-89529-399-4

Printed in the United States of America

10 9 8 7 6 5 4 3 2 1

Contents

Figures

Tables

Acknowledgements

I would like to thank Stephen A. Levine of the Allergy Research Group, California; Elaine Atwood, research officer of the Hyperactivity Association, South Australia; Ron Batagol, deputy chief pharmacist at the Drug Information Service, The Royal Womens Hospital, Melbourne; Dr Katelaris, consultant physician in Clinical Immunology and Allergy, Westmead Specialist Centre, Sydney; Anne Swain, dietitian at Royal Prince Alfred Hospital, Sydney; Betty Norris, National Health and Medical Research Council, Commonwealth Department of Health, ACT; Roger Sargent, Pesticides and Agricultural Committee, NH and MRC, ACT; Dr Jocelyn Townrow, Allergy Association, Australia (Tasmanian branch) and Dr David H. Allen, Department of Thoracic Medicine, Royal North Shore Hospital, Sydney. They have all supplied me with vital resource information used in the writing of this book. I would also like to thank Dr Stephen Davies, Biolab Medical Unit, London for invaluable discussions.

I am also indebted to Wendy for her ever ready assistance in the general preparation of the original manuscript.

Introduction

More frontiers of science have been crossed over the last hundred years than during the entire known history of human life on earth. As each barrier has been eagerly swept aside in science and technology, our enthusiasm has grown and our appetite sharpened as the next challenge presents itself. The most recent have been the space race and the 'Star Wars' concept of defence weaponry. This century we have risen to the demands of two world wars, and, more recently, the lure of accessible consumerism for all. We are now witnessing exponential growth in the fields of computer technology, electronics, physics, chemistry, biology, engineering and medicine.

We have also had our failures. Dams have burst, bridges and buildings collapsed, power plants exploded, air disasters have taken their toll, and more recently, the world watched in horror as an American space shuttle exploded in midair, killing all seven crew members on board because of a malfunction in one of the booster rockets.

Each new failure in technology has sent scientists back to the drawing-board for a rapid review of the situation: perhaps a replacement of materials or redesign of a component, before a much-publicised release of the 'Mark II" version.

This works just fine in the non-biological sciences. When faults occur, new material is used, a replacement part supplied, the circuitry altered or the equipment redesigned. We usually know about such faults almost immediately functional errors occur.

When we come, however, to consider the impact of the rapidly expanding chemical industry on human health the answers are not so clearcut, nor the solutions so easy. Over the last fifty years the chemical industry has supplied us with drugs, herbicides, pesticides, food additives and industrial chemicals.

While we are continuously exposed to these new agents either by inhalation, direct skin contact or oral absorption, we still know very little about the long term effects of such chemical exposures. Of greatest concern in recent years has been the steady rise in levels of food additives and chemical contaminants associated with our daily food supply. When a new chemical is directly introduced into it, or comes into close contact with our day-to-day activities, we try to get some idea of its toxicity by systematically exposing the substance to groups of animals for periods of time ranging from fourteen days to several months. The information collected on each chemical includes acute and chronic toxicity studies, the effect on the unborn foetus, and also any potential adverse effect on future generations. By using animals, we can speed up the expression of potential toxicity effects, since the life cycle of a small animal is substantially shorter than a human's. We can follow an entire pregnancy in a matter of weeks and observe the outcome of several successive generations of the same animal in a matter of months. There are also fewer ethical constraints involved in working with animals than when testing new chemicals on human beings. Such tests may involve the sacrificing of small animals and their litters after exposing them to large quantities of potentially toxic substances, but the whole area of toxicology and human exposure to chemicals in our food supply presently needs urgent investigation.

Classic toxicology places great value on an experimental procedure which examines the percentage mortality of a group of animals with increasing doses of a test chemical, the accepted value of toxicity being the dose that kills 50 per cent of the group of animals. This Lethal Dose is called the LD_{50}. Unfortunately the LD_{50} of a particular substance on a single species of an animal varies with age, sex, strain, diet, litter, temperature, and seasonal and social factors. The LD_{50} has been shown to vary more than a hundredfold between rats and mice, and differences have been shown to be sometimes even greater between these small animals and man.

Can we with certainty extrapolate the results of animal toxicology studies to the human situation? The answer is no. The organophosphate insecticide, maldison (malathion) is fatal in trace amounts for insects but is a hundred times less toxic for humans because we can metabolise the pesticide to a harmless metabolite, while the insect cannot. The reverse situation can also be true. We would not have had a thalidomide problem or the regular front page articles on birth deformities caused by certain drugs taken by pregnant women if there were any reliable method for assessing potential drug toxicity problems for humans. A chemical which appears to cause no immediate harm to the mother may harm the more sensitive developing foetus. We presently have no reliable test system that can accurately identify chemicals which are potentially teratogenic (cause birth deformities) or mutagenic (cause genetic changes which show up as birth defects in future generations).

All animal studies presently test a single pure chemical in a well-defined system of healthy test animals. This is not how it occurs in the human situation. There is frequently an exposure to small amounts of many different chemical agents over a considerable period of time. The total body load becomes of paramount importance because its detoxification mechanism may not be able to handle the cumulative load. Many of the chemicals or their metabolites are stored in fat tissue and are released during times of stress, weight loss and fasting.

We also need to examine more closely the effect of ingesting larger than normal quantities of food additives. Most studies on the effects of food colouring agents, for example, assume a daily intake of about 25mg, but a small proportion of the population is taking in excess of 350mg. The difference may be highly significant when toxicity is being considered.

Unlike selected groups of healthy rats, many members of our society are suffering from kidney failure and liver disease as well as inborn errors of metabolism. These people (predominantly the elderly, institutionalised patients and those suffering from other forms of illness) cannot metabolise chemicals as efficiently as healthy individuals. What is the effect of chemicals on them? Many chemicals are known to interact with drugs, food additives and food components in the gastrointestinal tract, and such interactions can cause an increased absorption rate and greater toxicity. For example, antibiotics have been shown to enhance the absorption of artificial colouring agents. Even vitamin C is known to increase the intestinal uptake of oestrogen from the contraceptive pill.

Modification of an originally non-toxic substance to a highly toxic analogue by the action of gut bacteria or digestive juices has also been demonstrated. In this respect a change in bowel habits towards constipation can cause a decrease in bowel transit time, with a corresponding increased bacterial conversion of procarcinogen chemicals, bile acids and other sterols (cholesterol-like substances) to carcinogens in the large intestine. This effect could be one of the major causes of colon cancer.

Studies presently examine the original chemical agent but there is good evidence to suggest that we should be looking more at the metabolic fate of a compound. Frequently it is the metabolised end product that causes the damage. Many biodegraded insecticides and herbicides are more toxic than the original substance.

We have yet to carry out studies which examine the potentially harmful effect of food additives and other food chemicals on human behaviour. Because of the great expense involved in organising such tests, and the real difficulties in finding suitable animal models, we really have no idea of the impact of most of our food chemicals on learning ability, attention span, emotional behaviour, IQ and many other related parameters.

So there are still many unanswered questions relating to the safety of food chemicals, and in recent years we have started to find strong associations between many common clinical disorders and specific food chemicals, findings which have given rise to renewed research interest in the whole field.

What is a food chemical?

Before examining adverse food reactions in greater detail, we should discuss what food is. Strictly speaking, food is made up of many biological molecules, all of which can be called chemicals. *Organic chemicals* are very large complex molecules that make up the bulk of our diet and include carbohydrates, proteins and fats, the three major food groups, called *macronutrients*. We depend also upon the *micronutrients* that accompany them. These are the minerals, trace elements, B vitamins, the fat-soluble vitamins A and E, vitamin C and other essential food factors such as beta-carotene, taurine and choline. All the macronutrients and micronutrients are essential chemical substances, which humans have consumed daily in their diets for thousands of years. It was not until recently that many of the macromolecules in our food supply underwent *chemical modification*. Such products include textured soy proteins, modified starches, polyunsaturated vegetable oils and low-fat, low-cholesterol dairy products, all of which may be handled quite differently by the body. We know that margarine has up to 30 per cent of the trans-isomer of fatty acids. This is a completely different structure even though it has the same chemical composition as normal fat. The body is known to react differently to this particular fat. When soy proteins or corn starches are modified chemically with acid, alkali and a number of different chemical solvents they change their tertiary structure. This means that the structural configurations of the chemically modified corn starches, soy beans, etc. that are presented to the digestive enzymes may be completely unique. The body may never have been exposed to them before and the long-term effects of consuming such high-tech foods are still not known. It is possible that many of the changes in manufacturing procedures may in themselves pose future problems to human health. (This topic is well covered by Ross Hume-Hall in his book *Food for Nought*, Harper & Row, 1984.)

There are many other small molecular weight chemicals that are also associated with foods that are far from beneficial. These are the naturally occurring *food toxins and drugs*, such as alkaloids in potatoes; salicylates in fruits and vegetables; theobromine in chocolates; caffeine in tea and coffee; amines such as histamine, tyramine, serotonin and phenylethylamine in cheeses, sausages, sauerkraut and fermented foods; serotonin in bananas and pineapples; oxalic acid in rhubarb; and a whole host of others which can cause pharmacological or toxic reactions in our bodies. In addition to these naturally occurring small molecules present in foods, we also have specific *food additives* which are put in because of their special properties. These include preservatives, antioxidants, artificial colouring agents, artificial sweeteners, flavours and so on. Many of these are identical to the naturally occurring food chemicals just mentioned, while others are not found in foods and are added after being synthesised in the laboratory.

Asthmatics have been found to suffer from increasing attacks and respiratory distress when exposed to some artificial food colours and preservatives. Patients with skin conditions such as urticaria and angioedema and children exhibiting hyperactive behaviour may be reacting to specific food colours, preservatives and salicylates, and require specially designed 'elimination diets' free of the offending agents. A person who suffers from chest pains, palpitations, burning skin, headaches or an asthma attack after a Chinese meal is most likely suffering from the 'Chinese Restaurant Syndrome', an adverse reaction to monosodium glutamate (MSG).

There is also another group of food chemicals, coming under the heading of *contaminants and residues*. These environmental chemicals end up in our food supply by indirectly entering our food chain. Sprays such as herbicides and the pesticides frequently used for crop dusting or on sugar cane or banana plantations or orchards can drift and end up contaminating food and water. So also can sprays which were never meant for the food supply, those that are used to control weeds in fields, for example, which may drift into catchment areas or be swept into the atmosphere and taken up into foods hundreds of kilometres away from where they were actually sprayed. Beef and dairy cattle are being increasingly quarantined as it is discovered that many of them are coming into contact with contaminated pastures and food crops. Sheep and cattle drenches are also indirectly transferring chemicals to our food supply. And many such as dieldrin, used to kill termites in the foundations of houses, can spread into the soil, contaminating plants and suburban hens fossicking among the foliage, the latter resulting in egg contamination. We also use aerosols in the home, the contents of which often end up in our food. So widespread is the pesticide/insecticide contamination of our food and drinking water through the biomagnification process, that penguins in the South Pole, birds on remote Pacific islands and native Australian birdlife such as the kookaburra and pelican are all contaminated.

'Safe levels'

Maximum residue limits have been placed on all foods in Australia, but the 'limited usage' laws placed on pesticides and herbicides do not appear to be working as effectively as some might have hoped. One reason is that policing the use of such chemicals is nearly impossible. We must now wait patiently for the slow biodegradation of residues of past sprayings and hope that common sense and wider education will prevail in future, and that people will start to appreciate many of the inherent dangers.

Heptachlor, a toxic metabolite of chlordane, is now found in 90 per cent of the population. The body fat of the average Australian contains two and a half times the amount of dieldrin present in the body fat of populations of other countries because Australians have continued to use the organochlorines while other countries restricted their use ten or twenty years ago. Another problem is that now the world sugar prices are dropping, ex-sugar cane growers are also experiencing difficulties. They are unable to grow alternative crops on their land, which has been heavily contaminated with organochlorine residues. Many other foods are also contaminated with residues of both organochlorines and organophosphates. In Britain over twenty years ago organochlorine residues were found in 25–50 per cent of the hard and soft cheeses, butter and infant foods analysed, and the situation has worsened since. A difficulty is that unfortunately, we just don't know what constitutes a 'safe level'; the maximum residue limits for food contaminants are based largely on the minimum detection levels of the measuring instruments, rather than known health criteria.

Other sources of food contamination which are causing great alarm in many industrialised countries are the toxic metals, mercury, lead and aluminium. Industrial wastes that are entering the atmosphere or streams and waterways can be the source of pollutants such as methyl mercury, a problem affecting many of the world's fish and shellfish. Mothers with high hair levels of mercury are known to be more likely to give birth to infants with congenital neurological abnormalities. Like MSG, mercury finds its way into the placenta during pregnancy and also to the infant through the mother's milk during breast feeding. Neither the foetal nor the neonatal kidneys or liver are fully developed, and as a result cannot efficiently remove the toxic metal, which tends to accumulate in the brain and other soft tissues.

It has also been found that lead in petrol is contaminating crops and cattle grown or grazing by the roadside. At present estimates, the lead levels in our food supply and lead stores in our bones are a hundred times greater than those existing in the pre-industrial world of 2,000 years ago.

While mercury and lead contamination seem to be prime suspects as causes of learning difficulties, emotional disturbances and inattentive behaviour in school children, aluminium toxicity has a high profile in many disorders of the elderly. High aluminium levels have now been associated with short-term memory loss; dementia; Parkinsonism; the motor neurone disease, ALS (amyotrophic lateral sclerosis); and even the brain tissue of Alzheimers Disease patients has shown aluminium accumulation. The greatest single cause of aluminium toxicity in the elderly is the daily consumption of antacid tablets. Nor does the infant population escape. A recent paper published in the *New England Journal of Medicine* has found that most infant milk formulas contain 200–300ng/mL aluminium, an amount sufficient to cause brain damage in children with impaired kidney function. Whether healthy children are similarly affected is not as yet known. Each year we gain a greater understanding of the importance of prenatal nutrition and dietary practices: we now learn that alcohol consumption during pregnancy can cause Foetal Alcohol Syndrome in the baby — a condition involving changes in physical appearance and irreversible brain damage.

Pregnant women who take low-dose vitamin and mineral supplements have been shown to have a lower incidence of offspring with neural tube defects such as spina bifida. This may be related to the prevention of subclinical vitamin deficiencies. A few extra antioxidant vitamins for neonates may also be a good idea in view of the discovery that it is now impossible to produce milk or baby food free from the organochlorine pesticides, aldrin and dieldrin.

Assessing adverse reactions

Any critical appraisal of adverse reactions arising from the ingestion of chemicals must examine all sources of chemicals in all foods. We cannot separate the chemicals that are naturally occurring in food from those that are directly added or exist as contaminants, particularly when many of the chemicals are identical in structure. Most people ingest several grams of chemicals each day, and many of them cause adverse symptoms in the unsuspecting. These can range from acute toxicity to hypersensitivity or pharmacological (drug-like) reactions. Some individuals may have been suffering from the adverse effects of these foods for most of their lives, but are still unaware of the problem.

It is obvious that we cannot eliminate our chemical environment overnight. But we can minimise our exposure to chemicals in our food and water supply, using improved knowledge of the sources of these and their potential toxicities. By the choice of selective diets and supplementary antioxidant nutrients we can also support our body's defence system, thus aiding the chemical detoxification process and reducing the incidence of adverse food reactions to chemicals.

1
Consumption of food additives

We have been adding chemicals to our food supply for thousands of years: to help us survive the long winter months without fresh foods, we found that we could preserve foods until the next harvest by using methods such as smoking, drying, curing, pickling, salting and adding a variety of local spices and herbs that prevented unstable foods from deteriorating.

Salt was used to preserve meat over three thousand years ago. Then, Mesopotamians were preserving both fish and cooked meats in fired clay vessels filled with sesame oil. In the Jewish community around 1600 BC the salting of foods was quite common. In the Far East during the time of Confucius (fifth century BC) soy sauce was used as a popular seasoning, and by 100 BC as a preservative.

We also found that the appearance and colour of food played an important role in our enjoyment of them. The ancient Egyptians used to colour their food yellow with saffron, and the Romans added chalk to grains so that the milling and processing resulted in a whiter and finer textured flour. By the Middle Ages we had become a little more sophisticated and started curing our meats with nitrates, and making cheeses using acid precipitation of milk or by the use of the enzyme, renin. Saltpeter (potassium nitrate) was added to meat to enhance its red colour and prevent it browning, and many meats were preserved in this way. During the eighteenth and nineteenth centuries copper was used to enhance the green

1

colour of vegetables. Between 1820 and 1860 reports of poisoning from the use of red lead and copper salts such as copper
arsenite, which was often used to impart a green colour to
desserts and cake icing, was common. Foods were also preserved with such toxic substances as phenol, creosote and
formaldehyde.

Artificially carbonated water was produced in Britain in the
1860s and food colours were legalised in the United States by an
Act of Congress in 1886. By the turn of the century cheeses and
butter were being artificially coloured, together with a host of
other commodities including sausages, noodles, jellies, flavouring extracts, ice cream, confectionery, cordials and alcoholic
beverages. At this stage there was no differentiation between
industrial grade dyes and food grade colouring agents. Up until
this time we had certain requirements of our foods relating
mainly to their appearance and ability to keep for an extended
period while remaining edible.

Over the rest of the century, all aspects of our food supply
have undergone changes of unprecedented magnitude, reflect-
ing the rapid growth in science and technology and major
sociological changes in Western society. The concentration of
populations in urban settlements, our fast-moving lifestyle and
changes in the traditional family unit, have all led to revolu-
tionary changes in agricultural methods, food harvesting, processing, packaging, storage and distribution. New foods are
now processed for convenience, quality control and cost
reduction as well as preservation. Consumers want foods that
look appetising, are easy to prepare, retain their freshness until
consumed, have acceptable and characteristic colour, odour,
taste and texture with a uniform appearance from one package
to the next, and have a long shelf life. They must be economical
to buy and geographically and seasonally available. Substitute
foods such as margarine, coffee whiteners and whipped toppings have appeared, while edible oils are now often substituted
for dairy products. Complex synthetic foods made out of
chemically crosslinked corn starch or textured soy proteins
combined with the appropriate food colours, flavours, etc., have
resulted in artificial cheese and extended meat protein products
which have reduced even further the price of major food items.
The importance of making everyday food products attractive to

the consumer by the use of colouring and flavouring agents, emulsifiers, stabilisers, thickeners, clarifiers and bleaching agents is highlighted by the United States Department of Agriculture survey on consumer lifestyle and food shopping behaviour. This showed that almost 40 per cent of shoppers were motivated to buy a product solely because of its *sensory appeal*. Another 32 per cent was more interested in the efficient use of time and money with the *price* of the product being of prime importance. Only 18 per cent was concerned with nutritional information, labelling, food additives and preservatives. Although many of us are unconscious of the fact, it is food additives that provide the qualities that most consumers value in foods. They help to:

1. *Maintain freshness and prevent deterioration*

Some additives protect against oxidation or rancidity due to chemical changes in a food. These agents are called antioxidants, sequestrants and enzyme inhibitors.

Physical changes such as emulsions breaking, lumps forming in a homogeneous fluid or water loss can be prevented by the use of emulsion stabilisers, anticaking agents and humectants. Agents can also be added to protect against spoilage or toxicity due to bacterial, yeast or mould growth.

2. *Amplify or promote sensory qualities*

Additives can impart colour, flavour, aroma, texture and improve appearance through the use of colouring, flavouring, sweetening, thickening and gelling agents, and the use of waxes, coating resins and carbonation.

3. *Facilitate handling or processing*

Additives occur as lubricants used in extruding, pelleting or other food-handling machinery, in dough conditioners, solvents, emulsifiers and antifoaming, anticaking agents.

4. *Maintain nutritional quality*

Vitamins, minerals and other essential nutrients are frequently added to foods to enhance and/or restore some of the nutri-

Table 1.1   Food additives used daily in the kitchen

Ingredient	Chemical name	Function
Vinegar	Acetic acid	Meat tenderising using a marinade
Egg yolk	Lecithin	Emulsifying mayonnaise
Cream of tartar	Potassium bitartrate	Stabiliser for beaten egg white
Garlic and mustard	Allyl sulphides and allyl isothiocyanate	Flavouring meat dishes
Vegetable oil	Linoleic and linolenic acid	Lubricant for baking, facilitating processing (dough expansion)
Egg white	Albumin proteins	Clarifying agent, stocks for consommé, binding agent (meat loaf), coating agent (deep fried food) and thickening agent (sauces)
Lemon juice	Ascorbic acid and citric acid	Antioxidant, preventing discolouration of fresh fruit
Sugar	Sucrose	Preservative antibacterial against mould and fungi, for jams, spreads, etc.
Honey	Glucose and fructose	Humectant and preservative in cakes and biscuits

tional value lost during food processing or not originally present in the food due to poor soil conditions (e.g. soil, crops and water in many geographical areas lack iodine, prompting the addition of potassium iodide to table salt which helps prevent goitre).

TYPES OF FOOD ADDITIVES

Chemical additives that are intentionally added to food can be grouped under six headings for discussion:

1. PRESERVATIVES, for increasing shelf life
2. COLOURING AGENTS, for improving appearance
3. TASTE AND ODOUR MODIFIERS, for enhancing flavour
4. TEXTURE MODIFIERS, for changing texture and appearance
5. PROCESSING AGENTS, to facilitate easy processing
6. NUTRITIONAL AGENTS, to maximise nutritional value

Preservatives

Preservatives are added to foods for two reasons; firstly, to inhibit unwanted chemical reactions within it after it has been processed and packaged, and secondly, to inhibit, retard or arrest the growth of microorganisms that are present in, or gain entry to, the food.

Antioxidants

As the name implies, these substances prevent oxygen molecules from attacking the food. For while oxygen is essential for life it has to be controlled by the complex biological systems in our body. The same applies in foods. If uncontrolled, oxygen reacts with food molecules which then become transformed chemically, destroying their original shape, structure and function.

The major types of antioxidants are effective in oils and fats because they can dissolve in them. They prevent rancidity by blocking or retarding oxidation or lipoxidation and the subsequent formation of peroxides and other reactive chemical species called 'free radicals'. These destroy the fat molecules. This results in a bitter taste, unpleasant flavour and odour, and, even more importantly, the production of potentially toxic or carcinogenic substances. The major fat-soluble antioxidants used in Australia and overseas are butylated hydroxyanisole (BHA), butylated hydroxytoluene (BHT), propyl, octyl, or dodecyl gallate, tocopherols (various types of vitamin E), tertiary butylhydroquinone and phospholipids such as lecithin. With the exception of BHT which is usually used in petrol, lubricating oils and rubber, these agents are added to edible fats and oils, margarines, dairy blends, salad oils, lard, dripping, essential oils, confectionery, dried instant mashed potato, walnuts and pecan nut kernels. (BHA and BHT are also used in the manufacture of clear polyethylene film for food wrappings and the amount of antioxidant migrating from the film to the food is not permitted to exceed 2mg/kg of food wrapped.) Most of the problems of 'oxidative rancidity' are now controlled by the food industry through the use of these fat soluble antioxidants. While many edible oils and fats contain naturally

Figure 1.1   Chemical structures of antioxidants BHA and BHT

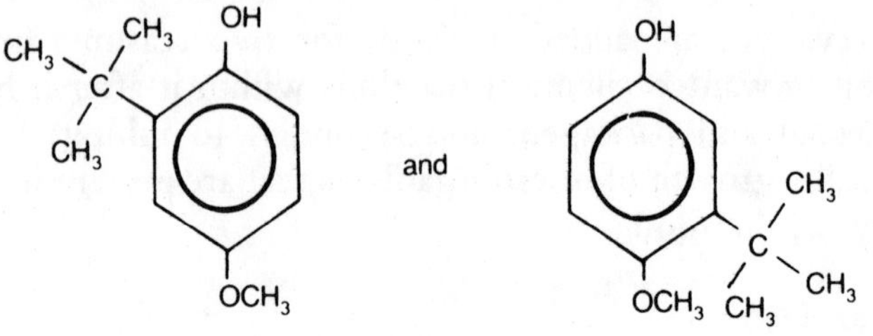

BHA (Butylated hydroxy anisole)

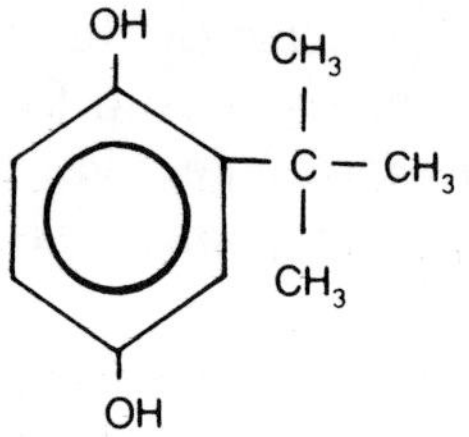

BHT (Butylated hydroxy toluene)

occurring antioxidants they are not effective at high temperatures and are present in such a small quantity (especially after losses due to processing) that they are inadequate for the necessary shelf life of the product.

Another type of oxidative change in foods involves enzymatic changes due to time-dependent activation of cellular and digestive enzymes within the food, leading to the browning of freshly cut fruit and vegetables and colour changes in processed meats. Fruits can be stabilised against such colour and flavour changes both during storage and on thawing by maintaining increased acidity: ascorbic and citric acids retard oxidative colour changes. Ascorbic acid, erythorbic acid and their sodium salts are also used as antioxidants in corned, cured, pickled, salted and cooked manufactured meat, frozen fish and frozen cooked prawns (shrimp).

The maximum permitted proportions of antioxidants allowable in the above foods as suggested by the National Health and Medical Research Council of Australia are shown in Table 1.2.

Antimicrobials

There are a wide variety of chemical agents which are added to
foods to control the growth of microorganisms such as yeasts,
moulds and bacteria. These have allowed a greater variety of
foods into the market-place, and also impart a longer shelf life
when compared with products processed by alternative
methods, including sterilisation, pasteurisation and cooking
which kill microorganisms, or drying, freezing or chill storage
which also prolong shelf life. We can also control the growth of
bacteria by dehydration of a food using sugar or salt and
changing the acidity to an unfavourable growth environment.

Table 1.2   Antioxidants permitted to be added to Australian food

Antioxidant	Food in which permitted	Maximum proportion permitted
Propyl (310), octyl (311), or dodecyl gallate (312) or mixtures thereof	Edible fats and oils, margarine, dairy blend, salad oils, lard and dripping	100mg/kg
	Essential oils	1g/kg
Butylated hydroxyanisole (BHA) (320)	Edible fats and oils, margarine, dairy blends, salad oils, lard and dripping	200mg/kg
	Essential oils	1g/kg
	Masticatory confectionery	200mg/kg
	Dried instant mashed potato	100mg/kg
	Walnut and pecan nut kernels	70mg/kg
Butylated hydroxytoluene (BHT) (321)	Walnut and pecan nut kernels	70mg/kg
Tocopherols (306)	Edible fats and oils, margarine, dairy blend, salad oils, lard, dripping and essential oils	No limit imposed
Tertiary butylhydroquinone (TBHQ)	Edible fats and oils, margarine, dairy blend, salad oils, lard and dripping	200mg/kg
	Essential oils	1g/kg
Phospholipids (322) (including lecithin) from natural sources	Edible fats and oils, margarine, dairy blend, salad oils, lard, dripping and essential oils	No limit imposed
Ascorbic acid (300), erythorbic acid, their sodium salts or a mixture of these	Corned, cured, pickled or salted meat, and cooked manufactured meat	No limit imposed
	Frozen fish	400mg/kg
	Frozen cooked prawns and frozen cooked shrimps	400mg/kg

In some cases we can control the proliferation of unfavourable bacteria using a controlled fermentation process, as occurs,
for instance, during the production of yoghurt. Here, desirable
bacteria inhibit the development of undesirable forms.

Many of the simplest antimicrobials have been used for
thousands of years and are still in common usage. They
include salt, sugar and acid, and the process of wood smoking.

However, for many foods these traditional forms of treatment, both physical and chemical, are inappropriate. Freezing,
for example, allows condensation to occur under metal lids,
favouring surface mould growth. Heat effectively sterilises the
contents of a can or bottle but after the container has been
opened microorganisms can enter. This problem becomes
significant when we consider that many containers are now
'family size' or otherwise large, and that a longer period of time
is required to consume their contents after opening. A further
consideration is that physical methods of preservation involving heating, dehydration and freezing require large processing
installation to make the technique economically viable and such
installations have a large and expensive energy requirement.

Raising the acidity of a food by the addition of vinegar (acetic
acid) or other acids is not sufficient to inhibit the growth of all
varieties of bacteria and is even less effective against moulds and
yeasts. Because of the recent trend towards foods low in sugar
and salt these two substances have also become unsuitable as
preservatives, as their reasonably high concentration is critical
for their antimicrobial activity.

These disadvantages have largely been overcome with the
introduction of the half a dozen or so major chemical preservatives presently in common use in Australia, Britain and the
United States. These are:

1. Sulphur dioxide and related sulphites

These are used to control microbial growth in low pH products
and to combat autolytic decomposition, auto-oxidation and
both enzymatic and non-enzymatic browning of fruits and
vegetables. Sulphur dioxide is added to wines, beer, cider, fruit
juice, mustard, preserves, dried fruits, dried milk, and dried
potato, to name just a few.

2. *Benzoic acid and its sodium and potassium salts*

These impart water solubility and have the capacity to retard and control the growth of yeasts and moulds, particularly *saccharomyces cerevisiae, aspergiller niger* and *penicillium glaucum*, as well as a limited range of common bacteria in foods which are acidic (i.e. below pH4.5). They are less effective on a comparable weight basis than sulphur dioxides and the related sulphite anions. Benzoates are added to carbonated drinks, fruit juices, cider, margarine, pie fillings, prepared salads and occur naturally in berries, prunes, plums, cinnamon and ripe cloves.

3. *Parabens*

These are chemically known as methyl, ethyl, propyl and other esters of 4-hydroxybenzoic acid, and are chemically related to benzoic acid, being most active against moulds and yeasts. The antimicrobial activity increases from methyl, ethyl, propyl up to the n-heptyl ester which is the most active. However, only the first three esters are permitted for use in Britain while the n-heptyl ester is permitted in the United States for preserving beer and a variety of soft drinks. They are also used in battered food (pastries, cakes, pie crusts, icing, toppings and fillings) as well as salad dressings, artificially sweetened jams, jellies and pre-serves and dried sausages. Parabens are not permitted as food additives in Australia.

4. *Sorbic acid*

Chemically called trans, trans-2 and 4-hexadienoic acid this and its potassium and calcium salts are effective against moulds, yeasts and many bacteria, and act as selective fungistats and fungicides for a wide range of organisms, including those producing mycotoxins. They are often more effective against yeasts and moulds than benzoates and like them, work better in an acidic environment, pH4.0–5.5. Sorbates are particularly useful for the manufacture of cheese and cheese products be-cause they destroy the undesirable lactic acid bacteria necessary for cheese maturation. They are also used in fruit drinks, beverage syrups, unsalted margarine, dried fruits, cakes, icing, and dips containing more than 85 per cent dairy products. Sorbates are used in Australia, Britain and the United States.

5. *Nitrates and nitrites (sodium and potassium salts)*

These are usually reserved for special applications. They are used in cured meats such as salami, frankfurters, bacon and bologna, to protect us against the lethal *clostridium botulinum*, the organism that causes botulism in humans. They also react with the myoglobin in the meats, thus maintaining the red colour. The only other permitted uses of nitrates and nitrites in Britain are during the manufacture of certain types of cheeses, but these do not include Cheddar, Cheshire, Cranapadana or Provolone types of cheese or soft cheeses.

6. *Propionic acid and its salts*

These are highly specific against moulds and fungal growth (fungistat) in bread, cakes and other flour confectionery. They are ideal in yeast-leavened bakery products because they do not affect yeasts, yet have good activity against the sporeforming bacilli that cause a condition known as 'rope' in bread. In the United States they are also used in pasteurised processed cheese and most economical cheese foods. Propionates have the distinct disadvantage of imparting their own flavours to certain products and are virtually inactive at pH values around neutral. For this reason their usefulness is strictly limited in Australia, Britain and the United States, though it has been suggested that they could be used to preserve wet grains such as wheat and barley.

7. *Nisin*

This is a polypeptide antibiotic produced by *streptococcus lastis*. It is a natural constituent of some cheeses and is used in clotted cream for the inhibition of *clostridia* and thermophilic spoilage organisms. It is also used in canned foods and in Australian canned soups provided the product is submitted to heat treatment sufficient to inactivate the spores of *clostridium botulinum*.

The use of antibiotics in foods is generally discouraged due to the present wide exposure of humans to subtherapeutic amounts of antimicrobials such as chlortetracyclin in beef and chickens and also to the overprescribing practices of many doctors, favouring the growth of new strains of antibiotic-resistant microorganisms against which we have no weapon. Nisin is an exception because it is rapidly degraded by digestive enzymes in the stomach and small intestines, minimising its effect on gastrointestinal organisms and ensuring that it is not absorbed into the human blood stream and tissues.

There are some other preservatives that have special purpose applications. These include biphenyl, 2-hydroxybiphenyl and thiabendazole, which are used in Britain for surface treatment of fresh citrus fruit at maximum levels of 70 parts per million (ppm) for the prevention of surface mould growth. Hexamethylenetetramine is similarly restricted in Britain to the preservation of provolone cheese. Formaldehyde is also on the list of permitted preservatives in that, under certain circumstances, it is recognised that it may find its way into food from packing materials or utensils, and also from its specific use as a preserving agent in the antifoaming dimethylpolysiloxane. In the United States, antimicrobial agents include fumigants such as ethylene oxide and ethyl formate which are used to control microorganisms and insects found on nuts, dried fruit and spices.

Colouring agents

According to the United States National Academy of Sciences, National Research Council, Committee on Food Protection, the addition of colours to foods serves several desirable functions:

1. It helps to correct for natural variations in colour or for changes during processing and storage;
2. it makes the food more visually appealing and helps emphasise or identify flavours normally associated with various food;
3. it assures greater uniformity in appearance, and hence, acceptability, by correcting natural variations and irregularities resulting from storage, processing, packaging and distribution; and
4. it helps preserve the identity or character by which foods are recognised.

Table 1.3   Artificial colours permitted to be added to foods in Australia, Britain and the United States

Shade	Popular name	No.	Permitted in			Countries banned	Adverse effects	Other names
			Australia	Britain	United States			
Yellow/Orange	Tartrazine	102	✓	✓	✓	Finland, Norway	Hyperactivity, urticaria, skin rashes, running nose, asthma, upper respiratory distress, cross-reacts with salicylates	FD & C Yellow No. 5, CI 19140, Food Yellow 4
	Quinoline Yellow	104	×	✓	×	Australia, Canada, Japan, United States	Safety unknown	CI 18965
	Yellow 2G	107	✓	✓	×	United States Under EEC review	Safety unknown	CI Food Yellow 5, Acid Light Yellow 2G, Acid Yellow 17
	Sunset Yellow FCF	110	✓	✓	✓	High safety status	Safety unknown	FD & C Yellow No. 6, CI 15985, Food Yellow 3, Orange Yellow 5
Red	Carmoisine	122	✓	✓	×	United States, Canada, Japan	Safety unknown	Azorubine, Food Red 3
	Amaranth	123	✓	✓	×	Austria, Finland, Greece, Japan, Norway, United States, Soviet Union, Yugoslavia	Possible teratogenicity	FD & C Red No. 2, CI 16185, Food Red 9
	Brilliant Scarlet	124	✓	✓	×	Canada, Japan, United States	Causes cancer in experimental animals	Ponceau 4R, Cochineal Red 4A, CI 16255, Food Red 7
	Erythrocine	127	✓	✓	✓	Japan (temporary)	Hyperactivity, sunlight sensitivity, overactive thyroid	FD & C Red No. 3, CI 45430, Food Red 14

Colour	Name	Number				Status	Effects	Code
	Red 2G	128	×	×	×	Under EEC review	As above	FD & C No. 40
	Allura Red AC		✓	✓	✓	Britain	Safety unknown	Food Red 17
								CI 16035
	Citrus Red		×	×	✓	Australia, Britain	Safety unknown	FD & C Citrus Red No. 2
Blue	Patent Blue V	131	×	✓	×	Australia, Canada, Israel, Japan, United States	Reduction in blood pressure, shaking, nausea	
	Indigo Carmine	132	✓	✓	✓	High safety status	Increased blood pressure	FD & C Blue No. 2
								CI 73015
	Brilliant Blue FCF	133	✓	✓	✓	Under EEC review	Safety unknown	Food Blue No. 1
								FD & C Blue No. 1
								CI 42090
								CI Food Blue 2
								CI Acid Blue 9
								Blue EGS
								Patent Blue AC
Green	Green S	142	✓	✓	×	Canada, Israel, Japan, United States	Hyperactive behaviour	CI 44090
								Food Green 4
								Lissamine Green
								Acid Brilliant Green
								FD & C Green No. 3
	Fast Green FCF		×	×	✓	Australia, Britain	Safety unknown	
Black	Brilliant Black BN	151	✓	✓	×	Canada, Israel, Japan, United States	Effects hyperactive children, asthmatics and those salicylate sensitive	CI 28440
								Brilliant Black PN
								Food Black 1
Brown	Brown FK	154	×	✓	×	Under EEC review	Suspected carcinogen: causes mutations in bacteria	Kipper Brown
								Food Brown
	Chocolate Brown HT	155	✓	✓	×	Under EEC review	Affects hyperactive children, asthmatics and those salicylate sensitive	CI 20285
								CI Food Brown 3

No other group of food additives has undergone such radical changes in the last eighty years as the colouring agents. At the turn of the century the United States selected food colours from some eighty different coal tar dyes; by 1980 only eight Certified Colours remained. These were FD and C Citrus Red No. 3 (Erythrosine), FD and C Red No. 40 (Allura), FD and C Citrus Red 2, FD and C Yellow No. 6 (Sunset Yellow FCF), FD and C Yellow No. 5 (Tartrazine), FD and C Green No. 3 (Fast Green FCF), FD and C Blue No. 1 (Brilliant Blue FCF) and FD and C Blue No. 2 (Ingotine or Indigo Carmine). Seven food colours were banned between the years 1956 and 1976 because of animal studies demonstrating evidence of carcinogenicity, mutogenicity or other toxic effects. In Britain the Colouring Matter in Food Regulations 1973 were amended in 1975, 1976 and 1978. Six artificial food colours were deleted from the permitted list which presently implements the EEC Food Colouring Directive, and with one or two exceptions there are no restrictions on the use of the remaining seventeen permitted artificial colours.

The total number of permitted colouring agents (including natural colours listed in Schedule 1 of the United Kingdom Colouring Matter in Food Regulations) is fifty-three. The artificial colours permitted in Australia and Britain are very similar and are compared with those permitted in the United States in Table 1.3. The three countries draw from a total of nineteen artificial colours. Australia uses thirteen, Britain sixteen and the United States, eight. The small numbers of remaining colours used by each country reflect not only the fact that animal studies have uncovered some very real potential health hazards associated with some of the deleted colours, but also that industry does not wish to spend huge amounts of money in carrying out necessary toxicological studies, so simply stops using the colour. In Australia many of the colours have been deleted simply because industry had no further use for them.

Of the relatively large number of remaining colours in Britain, it should be noted that lithol Rubin BK has had its use restricted to the rind of hard cheese only. Yellow 2G is likely to be deleted soon because the industry does not wish to carry out the additional toxicological tests requested, and Red 2G is only used in Britain itself (mainly in sausages) and not in other EEC countries. Green S is not a permitted food colour in Australia while Brilliant Scarlet, Yellow 2G, Green S and Chocolate Brown, permitted in Australia and Britain, are not allowed in the United States.

Identifying the colouring agents used in various countries has in the past led to much confusion because each country has had its own naming system. In Australia until recently the colour has been represented as the colour index number as indexed in the Society of Dyers and Colourists Colour Index. United States Certified Food Colours are represented as FD and C colours and numbers, and Britain follows the EEC E numbers system. As a result the blue dye called Brilliant Blue FCF has also had names and codes such as Blue EGS, CI Food Blue 2, CI Acid Blue 9, Patent Blue AC, FD and C Blue No. 1, E133 and CI42090. Fortunately this confusion has recently disappeared as Britain and Australia have adopted a standardised name and numbering system which for EEC countries is presently called E numbers, and will be introduced to Australia in January 1987. It will apply to all forms of food additives, not just colouring agents, and products containing food additives will have to state the specific name of each additive, or its code number, on the outside so that individuals with specific chemical sensitivities can identify the offending chemical and avoid the food.

A great variety of naturally occurring food colours is available to manufacturers, but few of them are widely used because they are relatively unstable compared with artificial colours and have a less intense colour. There is one exception: caramel. Ninety-eight per cent by weight of all colouring matter added to foods is caramel, and it is used in the colouring of spirits, beer, gravy, soft drinks and vinegar. The major commercially available permitted natural colours are listed in Table 1.4, together with the appropriate code numbers. Beetroot and chlorophyll are two examples of colours which are not very stable under food processing conditions. Chlorophyll can be stabilised, however, by replacing the magnesium atom in the middle of the molecule with copper to make the corresponding copper complex.

Table 1.4   Permitted natural colours

Natural colouring substances	Code numbers
Curcumin, Natural Yellow 3	
CI 75300 from turmeric	100
Riboflavin (vitamin B2)	
orange-yellow colouring agent	101
Cochineal (Carmine, carminic acid, Natural Red 4)	
CI 75470 extracted from the insect *Coccus cacti L*	120
Chlorophyll Natural Green 3	
CI 75810 Green extract from plants	140
Copper Chlorophyll Natural Green 3	
CI 75810	141
Caramel, also known as Natural Brown 10. Brown to	
black colour produced from sugar	150
Carbon Black (vegetable carbon) from combustion of	
vegetables	153
Beetroot Red (Betamin), Red colour from beetroots	162
Anthocyanins, water-soluble vegetable, colours giving	
shades of red, violet or blue	163
Natural Yellow 26, CI 75120 alpha, beta and	
gamma carotene	160a
Annato, also known as Bixin, Norbixin Natural Orange	
No. 4 CI 75120	160b
Capsanthin (Capsorubin), red colour from paprika	160c
Beta-Apo-8′-carotenoic acid Food Orange No. 6 CI 40820	160e
Beta-Apo-8′-carotenoic acid Ethyl Ester Food Orange	
No. 7 CI 40825	160f
Canthaxanthin	
Food Orange No. 8 CI 40850	161g
Titanium Dioxide Pigment White 6 CI 77891	
(used for colouring vitamin tablets and capsules)	171
Iron oxides and hydroxides CI 77472, CI 77499,	
CI 77489, CI 77491	172

Solubility is the main drawback for a more universal usage of riboflavin and the carotenoids (annato and its colouring principals bixin and norbixin) and beta carotene. These are essentially fat-soluble agents used in colouring cheeses and margarine. Carotenoids can be used for colouring aqueous solutions such as soft drinks but this involves the use of emulsifiers and gums to disperse the pigments. Carbon black derived from vegetable sources (not coal tar or petroleum products) is used mainly for colouring confectionery, and titanium dioxide is used to colour vitamin capsules and tablets and also to increase the opacity of sauces and for masking central colours in confectionery. Iron oxides and hydroxides are used to colour fish, meat spreads and pastes.

Table 1.5   Colouring agents used in Australian pharmaceutical preparations (approved by The National Health and Medical Research Council in October 1984)

Colour	Code number	Colour index number
Allura Red AC	—	16035
Amaranth	123	16185
Brilliant Black PN	151	28440
Brilliant Blue FCF	133	42090
Brilliant Scarlet 4R	124	16255
Canthaxanthin	161g	40850
Caramel	150	(Natural Brown 10)
Carbon Black	153	—
Carmoisine	122	14720
Carotenes (α, β, γ)	160a	75130
Chlorophyll	140	75810
Chocolate Brown HT	155	20285
Cochineal (Carminic Acid)	120	75470
Erythrosine	127	45430
Fast Green FCF	—	42053
(FD and C Green No. 3)		
(for use in CCNU capsules only)		
Green S	142	44090
Indigo Carmine	132	73015
Iron oxides and		77489
Iron oxide Hydrates:	172	77491
		77492
		77499
Lithol Rubin B (D and C	180	15850:1
Red No. 7) (for use in		
Laradopa tablets only)		
Patent Blue V	131	42051
Quinoline Yellow	104	47005
Saffron (Crocetin, Crocin)	—	75100
Sunset Yellow FCF	110	15985
Tartrazine	102	19140
Titanium dioxide	171	77891
Turmeric	—	75300
Violet BNP	—	42581
Yellow 2G	107	18965

Taste, odour and texture modifiers

Flavouring agents

There are over one thousand different flavour modifiers or enhancers which are presently added to foods either to enhance or reduce the taste or smell of a food. These small molecular weight substances may offer an additional sour or bitter taste or impart an aroma similar to fruits such as pineapple or passion fruit, for example. A combination of different volatile chemicals can even be used to impart the smell of fresh bread.

Artificial sweetening substances

For many people following low-calorie (joule) diets, artificial sweeteners are commonly used to replace the naturally occurring high-energy (calorie) sugars which include glucose, sucrose, fructose and lactose. These four sugars are present in fruits, vegetables, sugar cane and in the case of lactose, milk. The permitted artificial sweetening substances in Australia are:

1. Saccharin
2. Cyclamate (cyclohexylsulphamic acid or its sodium or calcium salt)
3. Aspartame
4. Acesulfame K

In Britain the only two permitted sweeteners that have E numbers are mannitol and sorbitol. Following a revision of the regulations in Britain in 1983 regarding permitted sweeteners, aspartame, acesulfame potassium, thaumatin and xylitol were added to the list. Hydrogenated glucose syrup, isomalt and saccharin are also permitted.

Emulsifiers

These are widely used food additives. When a processed food contains oil and water they will not mix, but with the aid of an emulsifying agent the surface tension at the interface of the water and oil layers is reduced. This allows an emulsion to form and is used in the manufacture of mayonnaise, margarine, salad dressing, soups, coffee whiteners, snack dips, and ice creams and other formulated foods containing dairy products or fats such as sausages.

One important area for the use of emulsifiers is in the bakery industry where moisture retention, volume, uniformity, strength and 'machinability' of dough can be improved. Emulsifiers reduce sticking and improve the texture of pasta products. They improve the shelf life of bread.

During the processing of dairy products, emulsifiers maintain stability and help the binding of starch to proteins. They maintain the fat droplet suspension in ice cream before freezing and facilitate the desired texture, smoothness and firmness while inhibiting large ice crystal formation during freezing. They inhibit the separation of fat and protein phases during the grilling of cheese sandwiches, cheeseburgers or baked cheese dishes, hence improving qualities such as meltability, spreadability and uniform flavour.

Without emulsifiers cocoa powder would not dissolve, processed meat products would lose much of their water during cooking, the fat content of chocolate would be much higher and the present trend towards producing low fat products would be impossible. The most commonly used emulsifiers are the mono and diglycerides, acetylated monoglycerides, lecithin, glycerol esters, polyglycerol esters and propylene glycol esters. Emulsifiers and modified starches permitted in Australia are shown in Figure 1.2. The proposed modified starches which have not yet been officially accepted in Britain also are shown in Figure 1.3.

Thickening and gelling agents

Thickening and gelling agents are necessary for the manufacture of many foods, including jelly, sauces, spreads, desserts, ice cream and gums and pastilles confectionery. The bulk of these modifying agents are naturally occurring substances.

Anticaking agents, sequestrants and humectants

A variety of mineral salts is used to facilitate the flow of finely divided powders such as table salt, vegetable salts, sugars, coffee whiteners and baking powder. These mineral compounds, notably carbonates and phosphates, act by preventing lumping, caking and the absorption of moisture (see Figure 1.4).

Other mineral salts and food acids are used to bind and remove unwanted minerals which cause undesirable changes in flavour, colour or turbidity and may reduce the shelf life of a product by accelerating rancidity. These agents are called sequestrants and are used to maintain the flavour and colour in canned food, spreads, mayonnaise and salad dressings. In the

20

Figure 1.2   Emulsifiers and modified starches permitted in Australia

Ammonium salts of phosphatidic acids
Diacetyl tartaric acid ester of mono and diglycerides
Glyceryl lactostearate
Mono and diglycerides of fat-forming fatty acids (471)
Phospholipids derived from natural sources (including lecithin) (322)
Polyoxyethylene (20) sorbitan monostearate (435) (polysorbate 60)
Polyoxyethylene (20) sorbitan tristearate (436) (polysorbate 65)
Polyoxyethylene (20) sorbitan monooleate (433) (polysorbate 80)
Sorbitan monostearate (491)
Sucrose esters of fatty acids (473)

Thickeners

Acetylated distarch adipate
Acetylated distarch phosphate
Bleached starches
Gelatine
Mono and distarch phosphate
Natural starches
Oxidised starches
Phosphated distarch phosphate
Pregelatinised starches and dextrinised starches obtained by chemical,
    enzymatic or physical processing that does not introduce a substituent
    group into the starch molecule or molecules produced
Starch acetate

Vegetable gums

Agar agar (406)
Alginic acid (400) and its sodium, potassium and ammonium salts (with or
    without modifying agents; calcium sulphate, calcium gluconate, glucono-
    delta-lactone), calcium alginate and propylene glycol alginate
Arabinogalactan (larch gum)
Carrageenan (407)
Gum acacia
Gum guar (412)
Gum karaya (416)
Gum locust bean (410)
Gum tragacanth (413)
Hydroxypropylmethylcellulose (464)
Methylcellulose (461)
Pectin (440a)
Carboxymethylcellulose (466)
Xanthan gum (415)

Figure 1.3   E Numbers for modified starches proposed for use in Britain (not yet accepted)

E1400	White or yellow dextrins, roasted starch
E1401	Acid treated starches
E1402	Alkaline treated starches
E1403	Bleached starches
E1404	Oxidised starches
E1410	Monostarch phosphate
E1411	Distarch phosphate ⎫ different production methods
E1412	Distarch phosphate ⎭
E1413	Phosphated distarch phosphate
E1414	Acetylated distarch phosphate
E1420	Starch acetate ⎫ different production methods
E1421	Starch acetate ⎭
E1422	Acetylated distarch adipate
E1423	Acetylated distarch glycerol
E1430	Distarch glycerol
E1440	Hydroxypropyl starch
E1441	Hydroxypropyl distarch glycerol
E1442	Hydroxypropyl distarch phosphate

Figure 1.4   Mineral salt additives permitted in Australia

Ammonium (503), sodium (500) and potassium carbonates (501) and bicarbonates
Calcium (170) and magnesium carbonates (504)
Calcium chloride (509) and oxide (529)
Potassium hydrogen tartrate (336)
Sodium (339), potassium (340) and calcium (341) salts of orthophosphoric acid
Sodium (223) and potassium (224) metabisulphites
Sodium and potassium polyphosphates (450)
Sodium and potassium pyrophosphates

Food acids

Acetic acid (260)
Citric acid (330)
Fumaric acid (297)
Lactic acid (270)
Malic acid (296)
Tartaric acid (334)
The ammonium, calcium, potassium and sodium salts of an acid set forth in this group

wine industry they are used to prevent turbidity due to the formation of insoluble metal tannin and metal phosphate complexes. Examples of sequestrants are phosphates, pyrophosphates and the food acid, citric acid. Some countries include the calcium and sodium salts of ethylenediamine tetra–acetic acid (EDTA).

Humectants are agents which are added to cakes and confectionery, to help them retain moisture, such agents are also added to marshmallows, desiccated coconut and cake icings. The two most commonly used humectants in Australia are glycerol and sorbitol.

Processing agents·

Some food additives are used to aid the manufacturing or processing of foods. These include dough conditioners, defoaming agents, anticaking agents, plasticisers, clarifying agents, enzymes and releasing agents. These compounds allow easier to manage, easier to machine or easier to recover finished products. Enzymes, for example, are used in the bakery industry to accelerate the hydrolysis of starch or in cheese manufacture for curd production. Releasing agents are antisticking, dusting, coating compounds, and lubricating oils or dry powders that prevent a whole range of foods from sticking to the containers in which they are prepared.

Nutritional agents

During food processing products undergo changes in acidity, temperature, light exposure and physical manipulation that result in the loss of micronutrients that were originally present in the food before processing. To offset the loss of some of these, selected vitamins, minerals and other food factors are often put back into the processed foods. Examples include breakfast cereals, bread and milk which may have extra thiamine (vitamin B1), riboflavin (vitamin B2), niacinamide (vitamin B3), vitamin A and D and iron added. Flours with added nutrients are called 'enriched'. Vitamin C is also added to many fruit juice drinks.

A complete list of all current food additives and their code numbers approved for usage in Australia is shown in Figure 1.5. This is generally similar to those food additives in common usage in Britain and the United States, where the list is based on the Food Additives Amendment of 1958, recognising three classifications of substances added to foods. These are:

1. *Regulated 'food additives'*. All new food additives must now be cleared via a petition to the FDA furnishing all information regarding established safe usage.

2. *Substances generally recognised as safe (GRAS)*. These are judged by 'qualified experts' as safe under the conditions of use on the basis of scientific procedures or common use in food. The criteria for GRAS exemption are based on the 'informal' use of scientific judgement by the 'experts' and often depends upon a history of safe usage of a food chemical. In 1973 the list included 553 substances for use as direct additives. See the following list in Figure 1.6 for some of the most common substances generally recognised as safe (GRAS) not including spices, natural seasonings and flavourings — leaves, roots, barks, berries, etc. — essential oils, oleoresins, natural extractives, including distillates.

3. *Substances with prior sanction or approval*. Many of these substances have been used in foods prior to the introduction of the GRAS list.

Figure 1.5   Food additives approved by the Australian National Health and Medical Research Council

Food additive	Number
Acacia	414
Acetic acid	260
Adipic acid	355
Agar	406
Alginic acid	400
Amaranth	123
Ammonium alginate	403
Ammonium carbonates	503
Ammonium phosphatides	442
Annatto (Bixin, Norbixin)	160(b)

Figure 1.5 (Cont'd)

Food additive	Number
Anthocyanins	163
Ascorbic acid	300
Beeswaxes	901
Beetroot red, Betanin	162
Bentonite	558
Benzoic acid	210
Beta-apo-8' carotenal	160(e)
Brilliant Black BN	151
Brilliant Blue FCF	133
Brilliant Scarlet 4R	124
Butylated hydroxyanisole (BHA)	320
Butylated hydroxytoluene (BHT)	321
Calcium acetate	263
Calcium alginate	404
Calcium benzoate	213
Calcium carbonate	170
Calcium chloride	509
Calcium citrates	333
Calcium lactate	327
Calcium malates	352
Calcium orthophosphates	341
Calcium oxide	529
Calcium propionate	282
Calcium sorbate	203
Calcium stearoyl-2-lactylate	482
Calcium tartrate	354
Canthaxanthine	161(g)
Caramel	150
Carbo medicinalis vegetalis (charcoal)	153
Carbon dioxide	290
Carboxymethylcellulose	466
Carmoisine	122
Carnauba wax	903
Carotene, alpha, beta, gamma	160(a)
Carotenoids	160
Carrageenan	407
Chlorine	925
Chlorine dioxide	926
Chlorophylls	140
Chocolate brown HT	155
Citric acid	330
Cochineal, carminic acid	120
Curcumin	100
Dimethylpolysiloxane	900

Figure 1.5 (Cont'd)

Food additive	Number
Dodecyl gallate	312
Erythrosine	127
Ethyl maltol	637
Ethyl ester of beta-apo-8′ carotenoic acid	160(f)
Ethylmethylcellulose	465
Fumaric acid	297
Glucono delta-lactone	575
Glycerol	422
Green S	142
Guar gum	412
Hydroxypropylmethylcellulose	464
Indigo carmine	132
Iron oxides and hydroxides	172
Kaolins	559
Karaya gum	416
L-Cysteine and its hydrochlorides	920
Lactic acid	270
Lecithins	322
Locust bean gum	410
Magnesium carbonate	504
Magnesium stearate	572
Malic acid	296
Mannitol	421
Metatartaric acid	353
Methylcellulose	461
Microcrystalline cellulose, powdered cellulose	460
Mono and diglycerides of fatty acids	471
Mono and diacetyltartaric acid of mono and diglycerides of fatty acids	472(e)
Monosodium glutamate (MSG)	621
Nisin	234
Octyl gallate	311
Paraffins	905
Pectin	440(a)
Polyglycerol esters of fatty acids	475
Polyglycerol polyricinoleate	476
Polyoxyethylene (20) sorbitan mono-oleate	433
Polyoxyethylene (20) sorbitan monostearate	435
Polyoxyethylene (20) sorbitan tristearate	436
Potassium acetate	261
Potassium alginate	402
Potassium benzoate	212
Potassium bromate	924
Potassium carbonates	501

26

Figure 1.5   (Cont'd)

Food additive	Number
Potassium chloride	508
Potassium citrates	332
Potassium ferrocyanide	536
Potassium lactate	326
Potassium malates	351
Potassium metabisulphite	224
Potassium nitrate	252
Potassium nitrite	249
Potassium orthophosphates	340
Potassium propionate	283
Potassium sorbate	202
Potassium tartrates	336
Propionic acid	280
Propyl gallate	310
Propylene glycol alginate	405
Riboflavin	101
Shellac	904
Silicon dioxide	551
Sodium acetates	262
Sodium alginate	401
Sodium aluminium phosphate	541
Sodium aluminium silicate	554
Sodium and potassium polyphosphates	450
Sodium ascorbate	301
Sodium benzoate	211
Sodium bisulphite	222
Sodium carbonates	500
Sodium citrates	331
Sodium guanylate	627
Sodium inosinate	631
Sodium lactate	325
Sodium malates	350
Sodium metabisulphite	223
Sodium nitrate	251
Sodium nitrite	250
Sodium orthophosphates	339
Sodium potassium tartrate	337
Sodium propionate	281
Sodium sorbate	201
Sodium stearoyl-2-lactylate	481
Sodium sulphite	221
Sodium tartrates	335
Sorbic acid	200
Sorbitan monostearate	491

Figure 1.5 (Cont'd)

Food additive	Number
Sorbitol	420
Stearic acid	570
Succinic acid	363
Sucrose esters of fatty acids	473
Sulphur dioxide	220
Sunset yellow FCF	110
Synthetic alpha-tocopherol	307
Synthetic delta-tocopherol	309
Synthetic gamma-tocopherol	308
Talc	553(b)
Tartaric acid	334
Tartrazine	102
Titanium dioxide	171
Tocopherol-rich extracts of natural origin	306
Tragacanth	413
Tri-ammonium citrate	380
Xanthan gum	415
Xanthophylls	161
Yellow 2G	107

Figure 1.6 **Major substances in common usage in the United States (GRAS list)**

Anticaking agents

Aluminium calcium silicate
Calcium silicate
Magnesium silicate
Sodium aluminosilicate
Sodium calcium aluminosilicate,
Hydrated (sodium calcium silico-
aluminate)
Tricalcium silicate

Chemical preservatives

Ascorbic acid
Ascorbyl palmitate
Benzoic acid
Butylated hydroxyanisole (BHA)
Butylated hydroxytoluene (BHT)
Calcium ascorbate
Calcium propionate
Calcium sorbate
Capryllic acid

Dilauryl thiodipropionate
Erythorbic acid
Gum guaiac
Methylparaben
(methyl-p-hydroxy-benzoate)
Potassium bisulfite
Potassium metabisulfite
Potassium sorbate
Propionic acid
Propyl gallate
Propylparaben (propyl-p-
hydroxy-benzoate)
Sodium ascorbate
Sodium benzoate
Sodium bisulfite
Sodium metabisulfite
Sodium propionate
Sodium sorbate
Sodium sulfite
Sorbic acid

28

Figure 1.6 (Cont'd)

Stannous chloride
Sulfur dioxide
Thiodipropionic acid
Tocopherols

Emulsifying agents
Cholic acid
Desoxycholic acid
Diacetyl tartaric acid esters of
mono- and diglycerides of edible
fats or oils or edible fat-forming fatty
acids
Glycocholic acid
Mono- and diglycerides of edible
fats or oils, or edible fat-forming
acids
Monosodium phosphate derivatives
of mono- and diglycerides of edible
fats or oils, or edible fat-forming fatty
acids
Propylene glycol
Ox bile extract
Taurocholic acid (or its sodium salt)

**Nutrients and/or dietary
supplements**
Alanine (L and DL-forms)
Arginine (L and DL-forms)
Ascorbic acid
Aspartic acid (L and DL-forms)
Biotin
Calcium carbonate
Calcium citrate
Calcium glycerophosphate
Calcium oxide
Calcium pantothenate
Calcium phosphate (mono, di,
tribasic)
Calcium pyrophosphate
Calcium sulfate
Carotene
Choline bitartrate
Choline chloride
Copper gluconate
Cuprous iodide
Cysteine (L-form)

Cystine (L and DL-forms)
Ferric phosphate
Ferric pyrophosphate
Ferric sodium pyrophosphate
Ferrous gluconate
Ferrous lactate
Ferrous sulfate
Glycine (aminoacetic acid)
Histidine (L and DL-forms)
Inositol
Iron, reduced
Isoleucine (L and DL-forms)
Leucine (L and DL-forms)
Linoleic acid (prepared from edible
fats and oils and free from
chickedema factor)
Lysine (L and DL-forms)
Magnesium oxide
Magnesium phosphate (di, tribasic)
Magnesium sulfate
Manganese chloride
Manganese citrate
Manganese gluconate
Manganese glycerophosphate
Manganese hypophosphite
Manganese sulfate
Manganous oxide
Mannitol
Methionine
Methionine hydroxy analog and its
calcium salts
Niacin
Niacinamide
D-Pantothenyl alcohol
Phenylalanine (L and DL-forms)
Potassium chloride
Potassium glycerophosphate
Potassium iodide
Proline (L and DL forms)
Pyridoxine hydrochloride
Riboflavin
Riboflavin-5-phosphate
Serine (L and DL-forms)
Sodium pantothenate
Sodium phosphate (mono, di,
tribasic)

Figure 1.6   (Cont'd)

Sorbitol
Thiamine hydrochloride
Thiamine mononitrate
Threonine (L and DL-forms)
Tocopherols
α-Tocopherol acetate
Tryptophan (L and DL-forms)
Tyrosine (L and DL-forms)
Valine (L and DL-forms)
Vitamin A
Vitamin A acetate
Vitamin A palmitate
Vitamin B_{12}
Vitamin D_2
Vitamin D_3
Zinc sulfate
Zinc gluconate
Zinc chloride
Zinc oxide
Zinc stearate (prepared from stearic
acid free from chickedema factor)

Sequestrants

Calcium acetate
Calcium chloride
Calcium citrate
Calcium diacetate
Calcium gluconate
Calcium hexametaphosphate
Calcium phosphate, monobasic
Calcium phytate
Citric acid
Dipotassium phosphate
Disodium phosphate
Isopropyl citrate
Monoisopropyl citrate
Potassium citrate
Sodium acid phosphate
Sodium citrate
Sodium diacetate
Sodium gluconate
Sodium hexametaphosphate
Sodium metaphosphate
Sodium phosphate (mono, di,
tribasic)
Sodium potassium tartrate

Sodium pyrophosphate
Sodium pyrophosphate, tetra
Sodium tartrate
Sodium thiosulfate
Sodium tripolyphosphate
Stearyl citrate
Tartaric acid

Stabilisers

Acacia (gum arabic)
Agar-agar
Ammonium alginate
Calcium alginate
Carob bean gum (locust bean gum)
Chondrus extract (carrageenin)
Ghatti gum
Guar gum
Potassium alginate
Sodium alginate
Sterculia gum (karaya gum)
Targacanth (gum tragacanth)

**Miscellaneous and/or General
Purpose Food Additives**

Acetic acid
Adipic acid
Aluminum ammonium sulfate
Aluminum potassium sulfate
Aluminum sodium sulfate
Aluminum sulfate
Ammonium bicarbonate
Ammonium carbonate
Ammonium hydroxide
Ammonium phosphate (mono and
dibasic)
Ammonium sulfate
Beeswax (yellow wax)
Beeswax, bleached (white wax)
Bentonite
Butane
Caffeine
Calcium carbonate
Calcium chloride
Calcium citrate
Calcium gluconate
Calcium hydroxide

30

Figure 1.6 (Cont'd)

Calcium lactate
Calcium oxide
Calcium phosphate (mono, di, tribasic)
Caramel
Carbon dioxide
Carnauba wax
Citric acid
Dextrans (of average molecular weight below 100,000)
Ethyl formate
Glutamic acid
Glutamic acid hydrochloride
Glycerin
Glyceryl monostearate
Helium
Hydrochloric acid
Hydrogen peroxide
Lactic acid
Lecithin
Magnesium carbonate
Magnesium hydroxide
Magnesium oxide
Magnesium stearate
Malic acid
Methylcellulose (U.S.P. methyl cellulose, except that the methoxy content shall not be less than 27.5 per cent and not more than 31.5 per cent on a dry weight basis)
Monoammonium glutamate
Monopotassium glutamate
Nitrogen
Nitrous oxide
Papain
Phosphoric acid
Potassium acid tartrate
Potassium bicarbonate
Potassium carbonate
Potassium citrate
Potassium hydroxide
Potassium sulfate
Propane
Propylene glycol
Rennet (rennin)
Silica aerogel (finely powdered microcellular silica foam having a minimum silica content of 89.5 per cent)
Sodium acetate
Sodium acid pyrophosphate
Sodium aluminum phosphate
Sodium bicarbonate
Sodium carbonate
Sodium citrate
Sodium carboxymethylcellulose (the sodium salt of carboxymethylcellulose not less than 99.5 per cent on a dry-weight basis, with maximum substitution of 0.95 carboxymethyl groups per anhydroglucose unit, and with a minimum viscosity of 25 centipoises for 2 per cent by weight aqueous solution at 25°C)
Sodium caseinate
Sodium citrate
Sodium hydroxide
Sodium pectinate
Sodium phosphate (mono, di, tribasic)
Sodium potassium tartrate
Sodium sesquicarbonate
Sodium tripolyphosphate
Succinic acid
Sulfuric acid
Tartaric acid
Triacetin (glyceryl triacetate)
Triethyl citrate

Synthetic flavouring substances and adjuvants

Acetaldehyde (ethanal)
Acetoin (acetyl methylcarbinol)
Aconitic acid (equisetic acid, citridic acid, achilleic acid)
Anethole (parapropenyl anisole)
Benzaldehyde (benzoic aldehyde)
N-Butyric acid (butanoic acid)
d- or 1-Carvone (carvol)
Cinnamaldehyde (cinnamic aldehyde)

Figure 1.6   (Cont'd)

Citral
(2,6-dimethyloctadien-2,6-al-8,
geranial, neral)
Decanal (N-decylaldehyde,
capraldehyde, capric aldehyde,
caprinaldehyde, aldehyde C-10)
Diacetyl (2,3-butandeione)
Ethyl acetate
Ethyl butyrate
3-Methyl-3-phenyl glycidic acid ethyl
ester (ethyl-methyl-phenyl-
glycidate, so-called strawberry
aldehyde, C-16 aldehyde)
Ethyl vanillin
Eugenol

Geraniol (3,7-dimethyl-2,6 and 3,6-
octadien-1-ol)
Geranyl acetate (geraniol acetate)
Glycerol (glyceryl) tributyrate
(tributyrin, butyrin)
Limonene (d, l, and dl)
Linalool (linalol, 3, 7-dimethyl-1,
6-octadien-3-ol)
Linalyl acetate (bergamol)
1-Malic acid
Methyl anthranilate
(methyl-2-aminobenzoate)
Piperonal (3,4-methylenedioxy-
benzaldehyde, heliotropin)
Vanillin

2

Hyperactive behaviour and food additives

Over the last ten to fifteen years there has been growing concern about the possible effect of food additives on behaviour patterns in both children and adults. It has been thought that many children, particularly, react to food additives by exhibiting hyperactivity, excitability, impulsivity and distractibility, tending to become unpredictable in their behaviour, and in a classroom situation exhibiting a high degree of irritability because they are forced to control or inhibit hyperactive tendencies. They may also exhibit antisocial behaviour. They have difficulties with other children, learning disabilities, low self-esteem and, often, depression. Hyperactive behaviour is found more in boys than girls, ten times more boys exhibiting it than girls. Parents may find their children have unusual energy and difficulties with sleep, often needing less than is usual. They have the capacity to wear out toys, shoes, clothing and even mattresses faster than other children. In the classroom they may find it difficult to get down to work or listen to or read a story. They frequently disrupt classroom activities, and often upset other children's play. Increased excitability often expresses itself as temper tantrums, aggressiveness, and a low frustration tolerance. Many hyperactive children slip behind in their grades. Their inability to get on at school often leads to their not developing satisfactory relationships with their classmates. Depression and low self-esteem may result if they continue to have failures in their relationships as well as academic disabilities (see Figure 2.1).

Figure 2.1

Symptoms of the hyperactive child

Marked hyperactivity and fidgetiness

constantly moving; runs, does not walk; rocks and jiggles legs constantly; touches everything and everybody

Disruptive, aggressive and excitable

behaviour is unpredictable: quick tempered, disruptive at home and school, panics easily, cannot be diverted from an action even when it may threaten life; low tolerance of frustration and failure

Short attention span

Unable to concentrate, learning disabilities, school performance not commensurate with IQ

Poor sleeping habits

Rhythmically pounds head on pillow during infancy; difficult to get to bed, finds it hard to fall asleep, easily awakened

Muscle incoordination

Exceptionally clumsy, may trip while walking, or collide with objects; problems with gross and fine motor movements in general

The California Association for the Neurologically Handicapped has estimated that the incidence of hyperactive behaviour and resulting learning disabilities has risen in the past decade from 2 to 25 per cent, in some cases as much as 40 per cent of an entire school population. Until recently, the most usual approach to the treatment of hyperactive behaviour has been via drug therapy with the most common agents being the central nervous system stimulants such as methyl phenadate (Ritalin) and dextroamphetamine. Surprisingly, these stimulant drugs tend to decrease such behaviour, and as a result of this, tend to increase a child's attention span. However, they have not been shown to improve learning ability, even though they markedly diminish disruptive classroom behaviour. It has been estimated that about half a million children receive some form of drug to control their hyperactive behaviour in any one year and virtually every psychotropic sedative and anticonvulsive-type drug has been tried on these so-called hyperkinetic children. Other approaches have included psychological treatment, such as behaviour modification, educational management, and family psychotherapy; behaviour modification, individual psychotherapy, family therapy and special education programmes have also been tried for the troublesome child. The problem with drug therapy is that the drugs have many side-effects which include headaches, insomnia, anorexia, nausea, stomach ache and depression.

As these children grow up, they tend to learn how to cope in social situations and how to control their hyperactivity. However, they take with them a deep sense of failure, very low self-esteem, a poor self-image and often suffer from depression well into adulthood. It is interesting to note that many alcoholics, sociopaths and depressives indicate that they have had histories of hyperactivity as children.

Most people have heard of Dr. Ben Feingold, the San Francisco allergist who first alerted people to the fact that food additives, particularly colouring agents, may be associated with hyperactivity and learning difficulties. Feingold first became aware of the relationship between food additives and behaviour after treating a woman suffering from acute hives in his allergy clinic in 1965. He guessed that the patient was sensitive to artificial colours and flavours and consequently withdrew them from her diet; her skin condition cleared up within days. Soon after, he received a phone call from a psychiatrist who had also been treating the woman for hostility, aggressive behaviour and difficulty in getting along with others. The psychiatrist had found that the woman's psychiatric condition had also dramatically improved, but that whenever she deviated from the diet Feingold had given her, her previous symptoms returned. Feingold has also noted that patients who react adversely to aspirin and other salicylates, by contracting urticaria or angio-oedema, also frequently exhibit mental symptoms including irritability and difficulty in concentrating. Many of these have only cleared up after aspirin and salicylates in foods had been eliminated from their diet.

Feingold noticed that there seemed to be a cross-reactivity between salicylates and other unrelated chemicals of the same molecular weight, such as tartrazine and non-steroidal anti-inflammatory agents including indomethacin. These observations prompted him to devise a special elimination diet for the treatment of hyperactive children. The diet was called the

Figure 2.2   The Kaiser Permanent (KP) Diet

Part 1   Foods containing natural salicylates

Almonds	Currants	Raspberries
Apples	Gooseberries	Strawberries
Apricots	Grapes or raisins	All teas
Blackberries	(Wine vinegar)	Tomatoes
Cherries	Nectarines	Oil of Wintergreen
Cider	Mint flavours	Bell peppers
Cider vinegar	Oranges	Prunes
Cloves	Peaches	Cucumbers
Plums		(pickles)

Part 2   Foods containing artificial colours and flavours

The salicylate containing foods may be restored following 4 to 6 weeks of favourable response provided no history of aspirin sensitivity exists in the family

Part 3   Miscellaneous items

All aspirin containing compounds
All medications with artificial colours and flavours
Toothpaste and tooth powder (substitute salt and soda or unscented Neutrogena soap)
All perfumes

Note: Check all labels of food items and drugs for artificial colouring and flavouring.
Source: B.F. Feingold 1975. *Why Your Child is Hyperactive*. New York: Random House.

Kaiser Permanent (KP) Diet (see Figure 2.2) and has been published in the book by Feingold, *Why Your Child is Hyperactive* (1975).

It was recommended that there were three areas of foods which had to be eliminated during this diet. The first group were all those containing natural salicylates; the second were foods containing artificial colours and flavours, and the third were miscellaneous items such as aspirin-containing compounds, and all medications with artificial colours and flavours, toothpaste and tooth powder, and perfumes.

After a considerable number of open trials had been carried out, Feingold presented his findings at a meeting of the American Medical Association in 1973. He related the sharp increase in the incidence of hyperkinetic behaviour over the preceding decade to the increased use of food additives and commercial foods, particularly those containing flavouring and colouring agents. He spoke of a dramatic improvement in the many

Figure 2.3   Adverse reactions to flavours and colours demonstrated by Feingold

Respiratory	Rhinitis, nasal polyps, cough, laryngeal oedema, hoarseness, asthma
Skin	Pruritis, dermatographia, localised skin lesions, urticaria, angioedema
Gastrointestinal	Macroglossia Flatulence and pyrosis Constipation Buccal cankers
Neurological	Headaches, behavioural disturbances
Skeletal system	Arthralgia with oedema

hundreds of children who had taken his additive-free diet and claimed that about 50 per cent of the children who undertook it showed marked improvement. These included rapid and dramatic changes in behaviour, children losing hyperkinetic behaviour patterns and motor incoordination becoming normal, as did sleep patterns. He also claimed that drugs that had been used to control hyperactive behaviour could be discontinued after two to three weeks of management of the special diet. There had also been marked scholastic improvement. Within a single term at school, children showed dramatic improvement in their reading and writing abilities.

Feingold had also noted that there were many adverse reactions induced by flavours and colours that affected other parts of the body. Adverse reactions were not just limited to abnormal behaviour patterns. Any part of the body could be affected, the respiratory system, the skin, the gastrointestinal, neurological or skeletal systems. These findings were published by Feingold in *An Introduction to Clinical Ecology* by Charles C. Thomas (see Figure 2.3).

Feingold made quite an impact with his claims and the implications for the food industry were enormous. As a result, many open trials were undertaken and results showed from 34 to 93 per cent improvement in children when they were on the special Feingold diet as judged by parents, teachers and paediatricians. However, open trials were subject to the major positive placebo effects of just the diet changes themselves, and it was claimed that many children described as hyperactive were in fact responding to their own or their parents' anxiety, which was alleviated, at least temporarily, by treatment which appeared to be complicated and powerful. Just the knowledge that some external factor such as an artificial flavour was responsible for the child's behaviour rather than some hidden organic defect reassured the whole family and caused changes in behaviour.

In early 1975 the Nutrition Foundation got together a group of nutritionists, child psychologists, psychiatrists, paediatricians and educators to examine Dr. Feingold's claims. As a result of this, many controlled trials were undertaken and the outcome of these were far less conclusive, usually showing that a smaller number of children benefited. There were several reservations raised at the time by critics of these trials.

For example, Feingold called attention to nearly three thousand different food additives; he said that the people who were performing the tests were really only testing one or two different ones, nowhere near the vast array which were eliminated in his diet. Of the three thousand additives, only ten dyes were tested. Most of the studies used doses of food colourings in the order of 2–26mg of colourings per day, 26mg per day being the Nutrition Foundation's estimate of per capita daily consumption of these colourings. However, the Federal Drug Administration admitted that the daily consumption of colourings is more like 59mg/day for children aged one to five; 76mg/day for children aged six to twelve; and the Gausian distribution curve showed that the 90th centile consumption figures were 121mg/day to age five and 146mg/day for ages six to twelve, with maximum consumption estimated at 312mg/day, far higher than the upper limit of 26mg used in the experiments. When another study (Swanson and Kinsbourne 1980) used colourings at this higher value, they found that there was clear evidence that the colouring-free diet led to a decrease in hyperactive symptoms.

Many other investigators alternated Feingold's diet with challenge diets containing the additive, and then reported the latter to have provoked no effects, or lesser effects than Feingold had reported. But the children who had been on the Feingold diet for a time tended to be healthier than the run of the

38

Figure 2.4   Food additives that the Hyperactive Children's Support Group recommend should be avoided

Tartrazine (E102)	Caramel (E150)
Quinoline Yellow (E104)	Black PN (E151)
Yellow 2G (107)	Brown FK (154)
Sunset Yellow FCF (E110)	Brown HT (155)
Cochineal (E120)	Benzoic acid (E210)
Carmoisine (E122)	Sodium benzoate
Amaranth (E123)	(E211)
Ponceau 4R (E124)	Sulphur dioxide (E220)
Erythrosine (E127)	Sodium nitrite (E250)
Red 2G (128)	Potassium nitrite (E251)
Indigo Carmine (E132)	BHA (E320)
Brilliant Blue FCF (E133)	BHT (E321)

Note: The Hyperactive Childrens Support Group was founded in Britain in 1977

mill hyperactive children who had not, and thus were more able to withstand the food additive challenge. Yet more researchers found that hyperactive children placed on a diet with no junk food for six months improved greatly on scales measuring hyperactivity, attention span and irritability. It seems that researchers should have distinguished between the Feingold diet fed ordinary children and normally malnourished hyperactive children.

Feingold's diet was specifically devised to remove artificial colouring, artificial flavours and natural salicylates. However, the tables that he used for determining the salicylate content of various foods have now been shown in many cases to be inaccurate. Using the latest scientific equipment, investigators at the Human Nutrition Unit at the University of Sydney have determined the salicylate content of three hundred and thirty-three foods. Most fruits contain fairly large amounts of salicylates, especially raspberries, raisins, prune and dried fruits. The blander tasting fruits such as mangoes, pawpaws (papaya) and pears contain less salicylates than the sharper tasting pineapples, oranges and berries. Vegetables varied in salicylate content from 0 to 6mg per 100gm of food (for gherkins). Some herbs and spices were also found to be high in salicylates. These included curry powder (218mg per 100g), paprika, thyme, dill powder, garam masala, oregano and turmeric. Eighteen different brands of tea were analysed, and most found to contain up to ten times as much salicylate as coffee. Cereals, meat, fish and dairy products were found to contain virtually no salicylates, and other safe foods for salicylate sensitive people include legumes, nuts and seeds in general. Using these values it is estimated that the salicylate content of the average Western diet ranges from 10mg to 200mg/day. The following figures (2.5–2.8) give the salicylate content of various foods. When preparing a low salicylate diet, choose foods from the 'negligible' table (Figure 2.5) and a maximum of three servings a day of food with a 'low' content. Actual salicylate values for each food can be found in *The Journal of the American Dietetic Association* 85, 8, pp. 952–8, August 1985.

Figure 2.5 **Food with negligible salicylate content (≤0.1mg salicylate/100g food)**

Fruit

Golden Delicious apple	fresh
Letona apricot	nectar
Banana	fresh
Packham (no skin) pears	fresh
Plum (Kelsey green)	fresh
Letona Bartlett pears	canned
Letona peach	nectar
Pomegranate	fresh
Tamarillo	fresh
Pawpaw	fresh

Vegetables

Bamboo shoots (Sunshine)	canned
Beans, blackeye	dried
borlotti	dried
brown	dried
lima	dried
mung	dried
soya	dried
soya grits	dried
Bean sprouts	fresh
Brussels sprouts	fresh
Cabbage (green)	fresh
(red)	fresh
Celery	fresh
Chives	fresh
Choko (Chayote)	fresh

Horseradish (Eskal)	canned
Leek	fresh
Lentil (brown and red)	dried
Lettuce	fresh
Peas, chickpea	dried
green	fresh
green: split	dried
yellow: split	dried
Potato (peeled)	fresh
Shallots	fresh
Swede	fresh
Tomato (Goulburn Valley)	juice

Condiments

Garlic (bulbs)	fresh
Parsley (leaves)	fresh
Saffron (powder)	dry
Soy sauce	liquid
Tandori (powder)	dry
Vinegar (malt)	liquid

Drinks

Aktavite	powder
Coffee (dandelion)	powder
'Ecco'	powder
Andronicus instant	powder
Harris instant I and II	powder
Moccona decaffeinated	powder
Nescafé decaffeinated	powder

40

Figure 2.5 (Cont'd)

Camomile tea	bag	Cottage	fresh
Milo	powder	Mozarella	fresh
Ovaltine	powder	Tasty cheddar	fresh
Cereals		Milk (fresh full cream)	liquid
		Yoghurt (full cream)	fresh
Arrowroot	powder	**Meat, fish, eggs**	
Barley	unpearled		
Buckwheat	grains	Beef	fresh
Millet	grains	Chicken	fresh
Oats	grains	Egg, white	fresh
Rice	grains	Egg, yolk	fresh
Rye	grains	Kidney	fresh
		Lamb	fresh
Nuts and seeds		Liver	fresh
Cashew nuts	fresh	Oyster	fresh
Poppy seed	dry	Pork	fresh
		Prawn	fresh
Sugars		Salmon	fresh
Carob	powder	Scallop	fresh
Cocoa	powder	Tripe	fresh
Golden syrup (CSR)	liquid	Tuna	fresh
Maple syrup (Camp)	liquid		
		Alcoholic drinks	
Dairy products		Gin (Gilbeys)	
Cheese, blue vein	fresh	Vodka (Smirnoff)	
Camembert	fresh	Wine, dry white (McWilliams)	
Cheddar	fresh	Whisky (Johnnie Walker)	

Figure 2.6 Foods with low salicylate content (0.1–0.5mg salicylate/100g food)

Fruit			
		Lemon	fresh
Apple (Red Delicious)	fresh	Loquat	canned
Apple (Mountain Maid)	juice	Lychee	fresh
Cherry (Morello sour)	canned	Mango	fresh
Custard apple	fresh	Nectarine	juice
Figs	fresh	Orange (Berri)	fresh
(S. and W. Kadota)	canned	Passionfruit	fresh
	canned	Persimmon	juice
Grapes, S. & W. seedless	juice	Pineapple (Golden Circle)	fresh
Grapes, Sanitarium light	juice	Plum (blood, red)	fresh
Grapefruit (Berri)	fresh	Rhubarb	fresh
Kiwi fruit	fresh	Watermelon	

Figure 2.6   (Cont'd)

Vegetables

Asparagus	fresh
Asparagus (Triangle spears)	canned
Beans, green French	fresh
Beetroot (Golden Circle)	canned
Carrot	fresh
Cauliflower	fresh
Eggplant (peeled)	fresh
Marrow (Cucurbita pepo)	fresh
Mushroom	fresh
Olive (black, Kraft)	canned
Onion	fresh
Parsnip	fresh
Pimientos (Arson sweet red)	canned
Potato white (unpeeled)	fresh
Pumpkin	fresh
Spinach	frozen
Sweetcorn	fresh
Sweetcorn	canned
Sweet potato, white	fresh
Tomato	fresh
Tomato, Heinz	juice
Letona	juice
Tom Piper	paste
PMU	soup
Turnip	fresh

Condiments

Bonox, liquid	extract
Coriander, leaves	fresh
Tabasco Pepper (McIllhenny)	sauce

Drink

Cereal coffee (Bambu)	powder
Cereal coffee (Reform)	powder
Coca-Cola	liquid
Coffee (Bushells Instant)	powder
Coffee (Bushells, Turkish style)	powder
Coffee (Gibsons Instant)	powder
Coffee (Harris Mocha Kenya)	powder
Coffee (Robert Timms instant)	powder
Herbal tea (fruit)	bag
Herbal tea (rose hip)	bag
Herbal tea Golden Days decaffeinated	bag

Cereals

Maize (meal)	dry

Nuts and seeds

Brazil nuts	fresh
Coconut (desiccated)	dry
Hazelnuts	fresh
Macadamia nuts	fresh
Peanuts (Sanitarium butter)	paste
Pecan nuts	fresh
Sesame seed	dry
Sunflower seed	dry
Walnuts	fresh

Sugars

Molasses (CSR)	liquid

Confectionery

Caramel (Pascall Cream)	dry

Alcoholic Drinks

Beer
Brandy (Hennessy)
Cider (apple)
Claret (McWilliams Reserve)
Sherry (Mildara Supreme Dry)
Sherry (Penfolds Royal Reserve)
Dry Vermouth (Buton)
Rosé (Kaiser Stuhl)

42

Figure 2.7 Foods with medium salicylate content (0.5–1.0mg salicylate/100g food)

Fruit

Apples (Granny Smith)	fresh
Apples (Ardmona)	canned
Figs (Calamata string)	dried
Cherry (sweet)	fresh
Grapes (Red malaita)	fresh
Grapes (Berri dark)	juice
Grapefruit	fresh
Mandarin	fresh
Mulberry	fresh
Peach	fresh
Peach (Letona)	canned
Tangelo	fresh

Vegetables

Alfalfa	fresh
Beans (broad)	fresh
Broccoli	fresh
Eggplant	fresh
Okra (Zanae)	canned
Peppers (green chilli)	fresh
Peppers (yellow-green chilli)	fresh
Spinach	fresh
Squash (baby)	fresh
Tomato (Letona)	canned
Tomato (Campbells)	paste
Tomato (Heinz, Kia-Ora)	soup
Tomato (Fountain)	sauce
Tomato (PMU)	sauce
Watercress	fresh

Condiments

Fennel (powder)	dry
Marmite (Sanitarium)	paste
Vegemite (Kraft)	paste

Drinks

Coffee (International Roast)	powder
Coffee (Maxwell House Instant)	powder
Coffee (Moccona Instant)	granules
Coffee (Nescafé Instant)	granules

Nuts

Pine	fresh
Pistachio	fresh

Confectionery

Peppermints (Allens Strong Mint) dry

Alcoholic drinks

Liqueurs (Cointreau)
Sherry (Lindemans Royal Reserve)
Spirits (Bundaberg Rum)
Wines Riesling (Lindemans)
Cabernet Sauvignon (McWilliams)
Claret (McWilliams Private Bin)
Traminer Riesling (Penfolds)
Rhine Riesling (Seaview)

Figure 2.8 Foods with high salicylate content (>1.0mg salicylate/100g food; foods with salicylate content >5.0mg/100g food are marked *)

Fruit

Plum (SPC, dark red)	canned
Prunes (Letona)	canned
Raspberries	fresh/frozen
Strawberry	fresh
Youngberry	canned

Vegetables

Chicory	fresh
*Cucumber (Aristocrat gherkin)	canned
Endive	fresh
Mushroom (champignon)	canned
Olive (green, Kraft)	canned
Peppers (red chili)	fresh
Peppers (sweet green capsicum)	fresh
Radish (red, small)	fresh

Figure 2.8 (Cont'd)

Tomato (Leggo)	paste
Tomato (Heinz)	sauce
Tomato (IXL)	sauce
Tomato (Rosella)	sauce
Zucchini	fresh

Condiments

*Allspice powder	dry
*Aniseed powder	dry
Bay leaves	dry
Basil	dry
*Canella powder	dry
*Cardamon powder	dry
Caraway powder	dry
*Cayenne powder	dry
*Celery powder	dry
Chilli flakes/powder	dry
*Cinnamon powder	dry
*Cloves (whole)	dry
*Cumin powder	dry
*Curry powder	dry
*Dill (fresh and powder)	dry
*Fenugreek powder	dry
*Five spice powder	dry
*Garam masala powder	dry
Ginger root	fresh
*Mace powder	dry
*Mint (common garden)	fresh
*Mixed herbs (leaves)	dry
*Mustard powder	dry
Nutmeg powder	dry
*Oregano powder	dry
*Paprika hot powder	dry
*Paprika sweet powder	dry
*Pepper black powder	dry
Pepper white powder	dry

Pimiento powder	dry
*Rosemary powder	dry
*Sage leaves	dry
*Tarragon powder	dry
*Turmeric powder	dry
*Thyme powder	dry
Vanilla essence	liquid
*Vinegar (white)	liquid
Worcestershire sauce	liquid

Drinks

Cereal coffee (Nature's Cuppa)	powder
Herbal Tea (Peppermint)	bag
Teas (all varieties)	bags and leaves

Nuts and seeds

Almonds	fresh
Peanuts (unshelled)	fresh
Water chestnut (socomin)	canned
Honey (all)	liquid

Confectionery

*Liquorice (Barratts Giant)	dry
*Peppermints	dry
Allens Kool Mints	dry
Minties	dry
Allens Steamrollers	dry

Alcoholic drinks

Liqueurs, Benedictine	dry
Liqueurs, Drambuie	dry
Port (McWilliams Royal Reserve)	dry
Rum (Captain Morgan)	dry

Figure 2.9 Low salicylate meal suggestions

BREAKFAST

1. Fruit salad from pieces of pawpaw (papaya), banana and peeled pear
2. A Golden Delicious apple grated with chopped raw cashews and fresh yoghurt (with juice of half a fresh orange, optional). Glass of Letona Apricot nectar or Peach nectar

44

Figure 2.9   (Cont'd)

3. For a high-protein breakfast choose lamb chops, eggs or lamb's fry. Season with garlic, parsley and small quantities of onion or tomato

LUNCH

1. Rice salad with salmon or hard boiled eggs. Season with garlic, parsley, celery, chives or soy mayonnaise
2. Chicken legs or salmon rissoles with coleslaw of cabbage, shallots, parsley
3. Bean salad with choice of borlotti, brown, lima and chick peas mixed with celery, shallots with home-made french dressing
4. Plain yoghurt with added banana or Letona peaches or pears

DINNER

Soups

1. Leek and peeled potato soup, thickened with cream (optional)
2. Split pea soup
3. Minestrone soup with borlotti beans, peeled potato, celery, tomato juice and mozarella cheese

Starters

1. Prawn cocktail on lettuce leaf using soya mayonnaise with small amount of tomato paste (Tom Piper)
2. Fresh oysters
3. Leeks vinaigrette

Main course

1. Lentil stew with celery, garlic, parsley, salt, Goulburn Valley tomato juice served with rice
2. Tuna rice casserole with grated cheddar cheese. Cabbage or lettuce salad with malt vinegar and oil dressing
3. Steak, chicken or pork with peeled potatoes, peas or brussels sprouts
4. Chinese vegetables, a sautéed combination of garlic, cabbage, celery, shallots, bamboo shoots and bean sprouts. Serve with rice and chops/chicken/scallops, etc. as desired, and soy sauce

Dessert

1. Banana on stick dipped in maple syrup and Milo, then frozen
2. Custard made from soy milk, egg yolks and maple syrup, served with peaches, pears, stewed Golden Delicious apples
3. Piece of pawpaw (papaya) with half a passionfruit

Many of the studies that were carried out to test Feingold's work also failed to recognise that there were other relevant variables that were not controlled: for example, Brenner in 1979 reported that artificial colourings and flavourings caused hyperactivity only in children with high blood copper levels. When twenty nine-year-olds who benefited from the Feingold diet were compared with fourteen nine-year-olds who did not, despite close adherence, it was found that their copper levels varied significantly: the ones with the high levels were not getting the same kind of positive results. It is also known that children in classrooms containing fluorescent lighting are more prone to hyperactive behaviour, so that this was a possible confounding variable and should have been controlled. When fruit flies were exposed to fluorescent lights after being fed yellow food dye, they all died of hyperactivity caused by exhaustion.

In addition, there is a tendency for many researchers to interpret positive data in a negative way. One costly program sponsored by the makers of Coca-Cola, Fruit Loops, etc., stated through the Nutrition Foundation that the results were unfavourable. In fact an editorial in the *Lancet* stated that in the preschool group all ten mothers and seven fathers rated their children as improved on the additive-free diet. In many of the studies compliance is the biggest problem. Children just will not stick to a special diet, and on frequent occasions up to 25 per cent of the parents involved decided it was just too difficult, and dropped out. Animal studies, on the other hand, confirm the harmful effects of food dyes. Compliance is better, because, unlike children, who frequently break their diet by sneaking the odd piece of food, or perhaps a chocolate bar on the way home from school, animals cannot. A study in 1980 by Goldenring, Wool, Schawitz, Batter *et al.* reported 163 per cent more activity and 128 per cent greater failure in avoidance learning in rat pups given small amounts of food dyes as compared with controls.

Similarly, many test tube studies show food colourings to damage nerve tissue. It has been suggested that much of the decline in academic ability that is exhibited in youngsters in the United States, Britain, Australia and other Western countries is due to the slow increase in the amounts and variety of food additives appearing in our foods (over the last ten to fifteen years).

Finally, many of the control studies used chocolate candy and chocolate brownies as vehicles for both the placebo and for the challenge with food dyes, because chocolate was found to mask food colour additives. However, recent research has found that 59 per cent of hyperactive children react adversely to chocolate itself.

Since Feingold's initial observations there have been enough trials carried out to show that at least some adverse behavioural influences are quite apparent in select groups of children due to the ingestion of food additives and colourings, and this tends to be confirmed by *in vitro* and *in vivo* animal experiments. But whether this effect is entirely due to the additive, and not to some other influence, is still not known. However, recent evidence suggests that the Feingold diet is in many respects inadequate because it looks only at naturally occurring food chemicals and chemical additives and not, for example, at the allergic effects of foods in general. What are the behavioural effects of ingesting eggs, dairy products or gluten if the person is allergic to one or more of these foods? The protein components in these foods can be partially digested to form exorphins (food components which act on the brain to change behaviour), or take part in the formation of destructive immune complexes in the body. There are many other mechanisms that have not been looked at by Feingold which are now under examination.

One recent study by Egger and Carter from the departments of Immunology and Child Psychology at the Institute of Child Health and Hospital for Sick Children in London looked at the effect of diet in the hyperkinetic (hyperactive) syndrome. A group of children were attending a special clinic set up to assess and treat hyperactive children by dietary means. Seventy-six children who had been diagnosed as either having hyperkinetic syndrome or overactivity as a predominant feature of a more widespread behavioural disturbance were selected for the study. In the first phase the children were placed on what is called an oligoantigenic diet for four weeks. This consists typically of two meats such as lamb and chicken, two carbohydrate sources such as potatoes and rice, two fruits such as bananas and apples, a vegetable such as brassica with water, calcium and vitamins. Those children who responded were then able to have foods introduced that were not included in the oligoantigenic diet, at the rate of one full serving at least each day; these were introduced weekly, one at a time. If symptoms recurred or deteriorated, the food was withdrawn. If not, the food was incorporated into the diet. Colouring agents and preservatives were tested by giving a subject three glasses of appropriately diluted fruit juice after excluding reaction to the fruit itself. Then sugar was tested, and if symptoms occurred with fruit squash, first tartrazine (150mg per day for a week) and then benzoic acid (150mg/day for a week) were given in capsules to confirm the response. Finally, a double-blind placebo-controlled trial was carried out on those children who were found to react to several foods and chemicals, and twenty-eight of the seventy-six children actually completed this test.

As a result of this trial sixty-two out of the original seventy-six children improved and a normal range of behaviour was achieved in twenty-one of these. Other symptoms such as headaches, abdominal pain and fits also improved. The double blind trial demonstrated that the symptoms returned or were exacerbated much more often when patients were on the active material than on the placebo. In this respect forty-eight foods were incriminated and artificial colouring agents and preservatives found to be the most common provoking substances, even though no child was allergic to just these. Colouring and preservatives caused reactions in 79 per cent of the children. Those who reacted to soybeans numbered 73 per cent; to cow's milk 64 per cent; chocolate 59 per cent; grapes 50 per cent; wheat 49 per cent; oranges 45 per cent; cow's cheese 40 per cent and hen's eggs 39 per cent. So there was a complicated interaction, not only with the chemicals, but also with (probably) the protein components of other foods. A full list of the foods to which the children reacted is shown in Table 2.1. The colouring agent, tartrazine and the preservative, benzoate, were the commonest substances provoking abnormal behaviour in the patients.

Egger found that many of the salicylate containing foods were in fact, at the bottom of the list. He claimed that the results of this study were not inconsistent with the largely negative results of the double-blind control trials of the effect of preservatives and colouring agents in hyperactive children, since

Table 2.1   Adverse reactions of hyperactive children to various foods and chemicals

Food	Number tested	Number reacted (%)	Food	Number tested	Number reacted
Foods universally tested			Peaches	41	3 (7)
			Lamb	55	3 (5)
			Turkey	22	1 (5)
Colourant and preservatives	34	27 (79)	Rice	51	2 (4)
Soya*	15	11 (73)	Yeast	28	1 (4)
Cow's milk	55	35 (64)	Apricots	34	1 (3)
Chocolate	34	20 (59)	Onions	49	1 (2)
Grapes	18	9 (50)			
Wheat	53	28 (49)	**Foods rarely tested and positive‡**		
Oranges	49	22 (45)			
Cow's cheese	15	6 (40)	Plums	9	2
Hen's eggs	50	20 (39)	Rabbits	6	3
Peanuts	19	6 (32)	Sago	5	2
Maize	38	11 (29)	Duck	4	3
Fish	48	11 (23)			
Oats	43	10 (23)	**Foods tested only in patients who reacted to antigenically related foods**		
Melons	29	6 (21)			
Tomatoes	35	7 (20)			
Ham/bacon	20	4 (20)			
Pineapple	31	6 (19)			
Sugar†	55	9 (16)	To cow's milk:		
Beef	49	8 (16)	Goat's milk	22	15
Beans	34	5 (15)	Ewe's milk	12	4
Peas	33	5 (15)	To wheat:		
Malt	20	3 (15)	Rye	29	15
Apples	53	7 (13)			
Pork	38	5 (13)			
Pears	41	5 (12)	**Foods to which there was no reaction**		
Chicken	56	6 (11)			
Potatoes	54	6 (11)			
Tea	19	2 (10)	Cabbages	54	
Coffee	10	1 (10)	Lettuces	53	
Other nuts	11	1 (10)	Cauliflowers	50	
Cucumbers	32	3 (9)	Celery	49	
Bananas	52	4 (8)	Goat's cheese	4	
Carrots	55	4 (7)	Duck eggs	2	

Note: * Given only to those who reacted to cow's milk.
　　　　† 5 reacted to both beet and cane sugar, 3 to cane sugar only, and one to beet sugar only. The parents of several other patients thought that large quantities of sugar provoked symptoms, without definite confirmation.
　　　　‡ Tested in <10 patients.
Source: Egger, J., Graham, P.J., Carter, C.M. *et al.* Controlled trial of oligoantigenic treatment in the hyperkinetic syndrome. *Lancet* 1:540–5 (1985)

these trials found that no child reacted to preservatives and colouring agents alone. Moreover, as previously mentioned, in at least two of the earlier trials, the placebo and excipient was chocolate, which caused symptoms in 59 per cent of Eggers' patients.

What these experiments tend to indicate is that salicylates are certainly not the only problem. Other chemicals and protein components of foods, or perhaps other biologically active amines occurring naturally in foods, might be contributing to the problem of hyperkinetic behaviour and, indeed, to other problems in children such as headaches, gastrointestinal problems, rashes, etc. Egger makes the point that of the sixty-two children who responded, 92 per cent of these were still continuing on the special diet when last seen, an interesting observation in view of the history of bad dietary compliance in past studies.

Anne Swain from the Department of Clinical Immunology at Royal Prince Alfred Hospital in Camperdown, Australia and Dr. Robert Loblay from the Human Nutrition Unit at the University of Sydney have also discovered that many food reactions in children are due to the whole range of naturally existing small chemicals as well as food additives, including salicylates, benzoates, nitrite, metabisulphite, propionic acid, azo dyes, antioxidants, brewers yeast, and amines such as tyramine, phenylethylamine, and monosodium glutamate. Most children going through their programs in Sydney react to between two and five of these challenge compounds. They point out that many of the reactive foods in Eggers' study contained significant amounts of natural salicylates, amines, and MSG, and in fact, the children were most likely reacting to these chemicals rather than to the protein components within the foods. They claim that the dose threshold for precipitating symptoms is lowered while children are on a restricted diet. Swain and Loblay find that sensitive individuals frequently react to several of these foods, particularly when consumed in combination or on several successive days. There also appears to be a dose threshold, and when the amount of the food consumed is great or the frequency of consumption rises, this threshold can be exceeded. It should also be understood that if many different types of food containing one particular com-

50

Figure 2.10   Food additives known to cause adverse reactions in susceptible individuals

Artificial colours

Allura Red	
Amaranth	123
Brilliant Black BN	151
Brilliant Blue FCF	133
Brilliant Scarlet	124
Carmoisine	122
Chocolate Brown HT	155
Erythrosine	127
Green S	142
Indigo Carmine	132
Patent Blue V	131
Quinoline Yellow	104
Sunset Yellow FCF	110
Tartrazine	102
Yellow 2G	107

Preservatives

Benzoic Acid	210
Calcium Benzoate	213
Calcium Propionate	282
Calcium Sorbate	203
Nisin	234
Potassium Benzoate	212
Potassium Metabisulphite	224
Potassium Propionate	283
Potassium Sorbate	202
Potassium Sulphite	—
Propionic Acid	280
Sodium Benzoate	211
Sodium Metabisulphite	223
Sodium Propionate	281
Sodium Sorbate	201
Sodium Sulphite	221
Sorbic Acid	200
Sulphur Dioxide	220

Natural colours

Alkanet	
Alkannin	
Annato (Bixin, Norbixin, Natural Orange No.4)	160
Anthocyanins	163
Beet Red (Betamin)	162
Canthaxanthin (Food Orange No. 8)	161
Caramel (natural brown No. 4)	150
Carbon Black (Vegetable Carbon)	153
Chlorophyll (Natural Green 3)	140
Cochineal (Carminic acid, Carmine, Natural Red 4)	120
Crocetin (Crocin, Saffron)	
Curcumin (Natural Yellow 3) from turmeric	100
Orcin	
Orchil	

Mineral Salts

Potassium Nitrate	252
Potassium Nitrite	249
Sodium Nitrate	251
Sodium Nitrite	250

Antioxidants

Butylated hydroxy anisole (BHA)	320
Butylated Hydroxy Toluene (BHT)	321
Dodecyl Gallate	312
Octyl Gallate	311
Propyl Gallate	310

Flavour

Monosodium Glutamate (MSG)	621

Note: Adverse reactions include behavioural disturbances, upper respiratory symptoms, skin disorders and gastrointestinal complaints, namely asthma, colitis, eczema, chronic colitis, hyperkinesis, migraine, rhinitis, conjunctivitis, urticaria/angioedema pound to which the child is sensitive is ingested on succeeding days then the threshold can still be exceeded. They further suggest that the interpretation of reactions to different food combinations is suggestive of pharmacological idiosyncrasy (chemical hypersensitivity) rather than food allergy. They have found that the incidence of reactions to food chemicals is similar in patients presenting with both urticaria and eczema, but the latter atopic group is frequently also sensitive to the common food allergens in milk, eggs, grains, peanuts and fish. They have found that these reactive foods usually do not provoke symptoms of hyperactivity or other behaviour disturbances in children so it would appear that the hyperkinetic learning behaviour problems that are experienced by children, are largely due to a reaction induced by small chemicals that either exist naturally in foods or are there as food additives or perhaps even food contaminants, but are not the result of more ortho- dox allergic reactions to protein or peptide fragments resulting in immunological reactions involving immune complexes (antigen-antibody) and other immunoglobulins.

Several animal and human trials have demonstrated that cer- tain behavioural effects can be elicited by ingestion of artificial colouring agents such as those found in food dyes. The two substances which have shared the limelight are Erythrosine, 127 (Red Dye No. 3) and Tartrazine, 102 (FD and C No. 5).

Erythrosine is a red food dye that belongs to a class of com- pounds called xanthenes, of which one of the members is the yellow-green luminescent dye, fluorescein. When four extra iodine atoms are added to the fluorescein molecule it becomes erythrosine. It is water soluble and about 20 per cent of the dye is absorbed across the gastrointestinal tract into the body. Appa- rently none is accumulated in tissues and the estimated daily intake is approximately 7.88mg/day for all reported ingested uses, including food, drugs and cosmetics. It is not degraded metabolically in the intestine in the same way as azo dyes, and its major path of excretion is via the bile. Less than 10 per cent of the unchanged compound appears in the urine after twenty- four hours. There is some evidence that erythrosine stains the renal tubules of the kidneys and a pink colouration of the urine has been observed with high-dose administration.

Because the bile is the primary route of excretion it appears that an enterohepatic circulation may be operating (i.e. the agent is reabsorbed through the intestines and recirculates via the bile), also indicating that erythrosine might accumulate if there were some blockage in the bile duct. The main adverse reaction to erythrosine appears to be its apparent association with impaired performance in hyperactive children.

Several studies have now shown that erythrosine can inhibit the uptake of dopamine (one of the putative neurotransmitters

Figure 2.11   Sensitivity to tartrazine (FD and C Yellow No. 5)

Tartrazine is widely used in food, drugs, beverages and cosmetics. Sensitivity to this colouring agent is largely, but not always, associated with aspirin sensitivity. About 15 per cent of those with aspirin intolerance react to tartrazine, and it is estimated that in the United States between 50,000 and 100,000 persons are so affected. Symptoms ranging from mild to very severe may be bronchospasm, urticaria, angioedema and rhinitis. Two researchers, R. Desmond and J. Trautlein from the Department of Medicine, The Milton S. Hershey Medical Center, Hershey, Pennsylvania, have expressed their grave concern at the prevalence of tartrazine in common commercial preparations and have warned sensitive individuals to be on their guard against this compound. The Food and Drugs Administration has called for the labelling of substances containing tartrazine. It is advised that consumers likely to be affected should read containers for the FD and C yellow No. 5 label before purchasing or eating these products.

The case history which prompted this report was that of a young medical student, aware of his sensitivity to antibiotics, grasses, moulds and so forth, but with no history of aspirin intolerance, who suffered tartrazine anaphylaxis at different times after eating a bright yellow commercial cheese product, three yellow jellybeans, and while receiving theophylline treatment during the jellybean induced attack. The theophylline and jellybeans contained tartrazine, but the composition of the cheese product was undefined. Two similar reactions followed the ingestion of different products containing the colouring. Symptoms during his attacks ranged from tightening in the throat, inability to swallow, profuse salivation and vomiting, light headedness, urticaria, to severe anaphylactic shock. The student was treated with adrenaline, oxygen, antihistamines and hydrocortisone IV.

In a letter to the *New England Journal of Medicine*, C. Ted Tse, from the University of Chicago Hospitals, Chicago, has listed some food products known to contain tartrazine. These include: orange flavoured drink mixes, ice creams and sherbets, gelatin desserts, salad dressings, bakery products, and some confections, especially those containing imitation butter, banana and pineapple extracts.

(This is based on reports in *Current Therapeutics*, 23: (1982) 56–7
and *N. Engl. J. Med.* 306: (1982): 682

of the brain) into animal brain preparations. This inhibitory action of erythrosine is consistent with the hypothesis that it can act as an excitatory agent on the central nervous system and is capable of inducing hyperkinetic behaviour. Another study has shown that although erythrosine given by injections at 50mg/kg to rats did not alter locomotor activity of controls; to 6-hydroxy-dopamine-treated rats, erythrosine at a level of 50–300mg/kg attenuated the effect of punishment in a conflict paradigm. Yet another paper has examined the neurotransmitter release from a vertebrate neuromuscular synapse and how it was affected by erythrosine. When the dye was applied to isolated neuromuscular synapses in a frog, its effect on the spontaneous release of acetyl choline (one of the major chemicals for transmitting nerve impulses to the muscles) was examined with electrophysiological techniques. At concentrations of 10 mmol or greater this dye produced an irreversible dose-dependent increase in neurotransmitter release.

All these animal studies so far, then, have suggested that erythrosine inhibits the uptake of dopamine, choline, GABA, glycine, glutamate and noradrenaline — all important chemical messengers for conveying information from one part of the brain to the other, or for transferring information from the brain to the muscles of the body.

Some studies, however, have suggested that erythrosine has great difficulty in actually crossing the blood-brain barrier, the biological barrier between the blood and the brain which prevents unwanted substances gaining entry, in any significant amounts. It is suggested that erythrosine may act to modulate molecular events such as the inflow and outflow of various organic acids, ions, or neurochemical precursors, at the blood-brain barrier itself. However, there is another mechanism that is gaining more recognition of late. Experiments with rats have shown that erythrosine delivered to the stomach by intubation has caused anaemia, hypercholesterolaemia (raised blood levels of cholesterol) and elevation in protein-bound-iodine (PBI). Other studies using mini-pigs have demonstrated a dose-related thyroid effect which included changes in the thyroid hormones thyroxin (T_4), triiodothyronine (T_3) and protein bound iodine after erythrosine ingestion at 167–1500mg/kg/day. These studies with mini-pigs showed that as much as 50 per cent of the ingested dose of erythrosine was absorbed, and was able to influence thyroxin levels, thyroid uptake and thyroid-iodine retention. Radioactive erythrosine first appeared in the liver and later was found in the thyroid gland itself and maximum levels were reached in about two weeks. It is possible that erythrosine may in fact induce a form of hyperthyroidism that can cause symptoms such as hyperactivity, irritability and emotional lability. While large doses of erythrosine have certainly been associated with increases in iodine uptake by the thyroid gland, the erythrosine ingested by humans, either in the diet or in drug capsules, has been associated only with serum elevations of protein-bound-iodine. It has been suggested that smaller doses of erythrosine may enhance the uptake of iodine into the thyroid gland.

Dr. John Hattan and others from the Food and Drug Administration in Washington suggest that minor alterations in thyroid function may be manifested as behavioural changes, especially in settings of environmental change. They propose that a delicate neurological balance in susceptible individuals may be altered by factors that influence the fine tuning of thyroid hormone homeostasis, and although no evidence exists at present this would indicate that erythrosine can act in this capacity. It is possible to hypothesise that because of its structural similarity with thyroxin, erythrosine might act in a manner analogous to that of thyroxin. Erythrosine has actually been shown to bind and migrate with the same type of proteins in the bloodstream as thyroxin. Hattan and his co-workers hypothesise that the hyperactivity changes related to the thyroid gland may occur because erythrosine either displaces thyroxin from protein-binding sites or interferes with thyroxin activity (by feedback or metabolism), or alters thyroxin-dependent neuronal receptor populations. Further studies along this line may prove very interesting.

While food colours and food additives have been implicated for a long time as a major cause of hyperactivity other factors in the environment may also be responsible for hyperactive behaviour. Many patients are not only food and chemical sensitive, but also react to atmospheric pollutions. These are chemicals in the air around us. Both foodborne and atmospheric chemicals act together in children. Joseph McGovern, a specialist in the field of allergy and clinical ecology, practises in Oakland, California, and has found that three-quarters of hyperactive children can be shown to be petrochemically sensitive. The major chemical excitants include hydrocarbons, petrol, diesel fumes, outgassing paints, formaldehyde and aerosols. McGovern claims that the cerebrum, which is the thinking part of our brain, is often the first major organ system to react to chemicals found in the environment. The problem is more intricately defined by the role of certain neurotransmitters, all of which are balanced in a delicate equilibrium in normal individuals. The compensatory feedback mechanisms between the brain neurotransmitters, dopamine, serotonin, noradrenaline and acetylcholine can be easily disturbed in persons with sensitivities to atmospheric hydrocarbons.

McGovern recently set up a scientifically controlled study using thirteen hyperactive children in order to study the relationship between naturally occurring food compounds and hyperkinetic reactions in children with food allergies. The children were studied under double-blind placebo control conditions and were challenged with eight common foods, thirteen phenolic compounds and many of the traditional allergenic substances such as dog dander and house dust. The following substances, listed in descending order, were found to be most frequently provokers of hyperkinesis: salicylates, ethanol, dopamine, noradrenaline, histamine, coumarin, indole, ascorbic acid, gallic acid, phenylisothiocyanate, phenylalanine and uric acid (see Table 2.2). They are low molecular weight compounds occurring in foods, that usually have an aromatic ring structure, often with phenolic hydroxyls. McGovern found that 57 per cent of hyperactive children reacted adversely to challenge testing with phenolic neurotransmitters. All patients tested who became hyperactive had some immunological abnormalities in the blood, and the typical profile included depressed serotonin, elevated histamine and prostaglandins, with abnormal complement and immune complex formation. These changes in the blood chemistry are characteristic of a person suffering from immune malfunction. Other work has shown that experimental animals exposed to these aromatic substances exhibit evidence of immune suppression, especially a dramatic drop in a certain subgroup of T-lymphocytes

Table 2.2   Relative frequency of hyperkinetic reactions induced by provocative tests

Substance tested	Frequency of positive response
Acetyl salicylate (aspirin)	80%
Ethanol	70%
Dopamine, Norepinephrine, Histamine	50%
Coumarin	40%
Indole	36%
Malvin, Ascorbic acid, Gallic acid	33%
Sugar, Phenyl isothiocyanate, Phenylalanine	30%
Corn, beef, eggs, Uric acid	25%
Cat hair, house dust	25%
Dog dander	10%

Note: 13 patients challenged with an average of 32 allergenic extracts or chemical solutions; each patient sustained an average of 7 hyperkinetic reactions.

Source: McGovern, J.J., Gardener, R.W., Painter, K. *et al.* Natural foodborne aromatics induce behavioural disturbances in children with hyperkinesis. *Int. J. Biosocial Research* 4(1): 40–2 (1983).

called T–suppressor cells or in total lymphocyte cell numbers.

Experiments have found that if animals are continuously exposed to phenols and other aromatic compounds, eventually the other group of T–lymphocytes called T–helper cells become depressed and animals lose their immune competency. McGovern has found that these reactions are also induced in humans by foodborne phenols and atmospheric pollutants. There are two phases of activity when a reactive chemical is exposed to a potentially hyperkinetic subject. Firstly, there is an agitation phase where physical hyperactivity is obvious and then there is an attention span deficit. Repeated exposure orally of small doses of the chemical reliably produces the hyperactivity syndrome, with mental and physical excitement and within a few minutes, the inverse phenomenon usually occurs. The child then becomes withdrawn, depressed and sleepy and finally falls asleep. In other words, there is a stimulatory and a depressed phase in the same person, often due to an exposure to different amounts of the same chemical.

McGovern feels that the underlying cause of hyperkinesis may be a defect in dopamine (one of the brain's chemical messengers) metabolism, which may be acquired or inherited, and he notes that two other well-known disorders related to disregulation of dopamine metabolism are schizophrenia and

Parkinson's Disease. When patients with schizophrenia or Parkinson's Disease have been examined, it was found that many of them are also allergic or hypersensitive to foods and chemicals.

We might well ask how it is that so many of these chemicals which can cause such bad effects are allowed to appear in our daily food supply with such monotonous regularity. To answer this question we need to look at the present screening process for new food additives. Originally some of these, such as colours, flavours and preservatives were regulated, and indeed many of the chemicals presently in our foods have been there for many, many years. However, in recent times there are three criteria that are considered before a new chemical is introduced into our food system. Firstly, what is the acute toxicity of the substance? Secondly, does it have mutagenic properties (affecting future generations) or teratogenic ones (affecting the foetus)? Thirdly, is the substance carcinogenic, or cancer producing? It is fairly easy to test whether a substance is going to be toxic in one of the organs such as the liver, kidney or bone marrow, but such tests do not screen agents for potential long-term hazardous effects due to cumulative low-dose administration, or to subtle changes that are not looked for in normal toxicological testing, such as behavioural effects.

In eastern Europe, and especially in the Soviet Union, toxicology also includes the effect of a chemical on animal behaviour. However, this form of testing has never been applied in the West, so a food additive can have an adverse effect on behaviour and still get through the normal screening process. The reason that these tests are not routinely performed is that they are difficult to conduct, and the behaviour of man differs so greatly from animals that there are serious questions as to whether or not animal models can be established. Also, if one is concerned with the behavioural toxicity of agents administered in low doses for long periods of time, the costs of such tests would be prohibitive. So all the common food flavours, colours and preservatives are looked on as safe simply because they are not carcinogenic and have not been shown to cause any organic pathology, including death, in doses that are much higher than those which humans normally consume in the short term.

One of the major problems with testing food additives on

58

Figure 2.12   Examples of the three major chemical structures used to produce synthetic food colours

AZO DYES   (– N = N –) reds, oranges, black brown and yellows

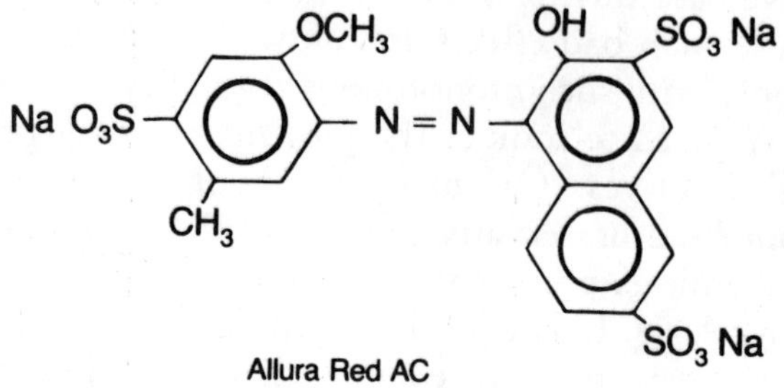

Other examples:
Amaranth
Brilliant Scarlet 4R
Carmoisine
Chlorazol pink
Sunset yellow
Tartrazine
Yellow 2G

Allura Red AC

TRIPHENYLENE DYES (Ph – C $\stackrel{Ph}{\underset{Ph}{<}}$)   green, blue and violet

other examples:
Brilliant blue FCF

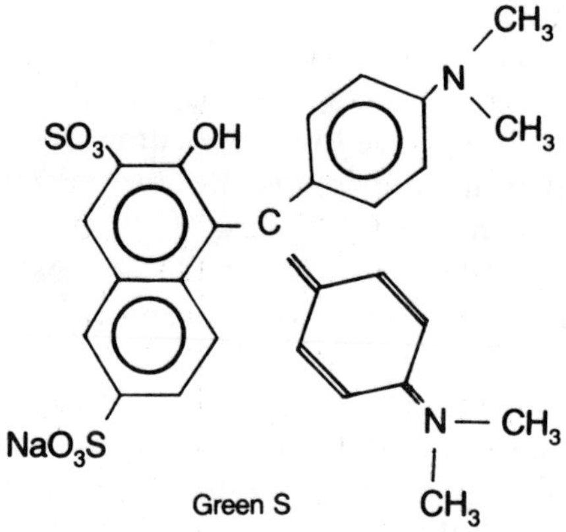

Green S

XANTHENE

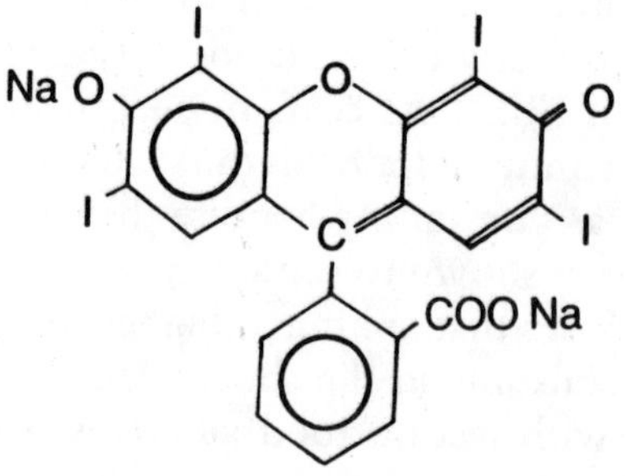

ERYTHROSINE

animals is the marked species differences related to absorption, metabolism and toxicity. A good example is erythrosine — while this colouring agent was found to be relatively non-toxic in rodents at a level of 160–170mg/kg/day, the same agent tested in mini-pigs was found to adversely affect thyroid function, causing decreases in serum levels of the thyroid hormone, thyroxin, even at very small levels.

It is also very difficult to evaluate the effects of ingestion of a single compound because it may be changed into several different ones in the gastrointestinal tract before it is absorbed. For example, many of the water-soluble food colours that are presently on the market are in fact aromatic sulphonic acid derivatives such as tartrazine, where aromatic sulphonic acid groups are linked by an azo group to another aromatic sulphonic acid (see Figure 2.13). The absorption and excretion of these water-soluble azo dyes are altered by their primary metabolism via gut bacteria which split the azo group. There is always the possibility that one of these metabolites arising from splitting the azo group may interact with other dietary constituents in the human diet.

Animal studies have shown that while most of the red and yellow dyes are found in the faeces of treated animals in the order of about 2 per cent, if an animal has been pretreated with antibiotics, then nearly 10 per cent of the administered dose of a red dye such as Red Dye No. 2 has been found in the faeces. An earlier study of the excretion and metabolism of edible food dyes by Daniel (1962), who studied tartrazine, sunset yellow and erythrosine, indicated that erythrosine was eliminated in at least 60–70 per cent yield directly in the faeces, with a small amount coming from the bile. However, with the two azo dyes, tartrazine and sunset yellow, Daniel found less than 2 per cent of either excreted in the urine, with most of the material appearing in urine or bile as various metabolites. These included sulphonilic acid, which accounted for more than 50 per cent of both dyes, and acetomethdobenzensulphonic acid which accounted for approximately 20 per cent. Other metabolites were found arising from sunset yellow.

One of the biggest problems in extrapolating the results of animal studies to the human situation is the inability to evaluate the interactions between the additives such as food colours and other dietary constituents, drugs and food contaminants. It is now known, for example, that tartrazine interacts directly with a substance called DSS, dioptilsodiumsulphosuccinate, which is widely used as a faecal softening agent in laxatives and other pharmaceuticals. When the tartrazine and DSS are administered together there is an inhibition of the metabolism of the tartrazine by intestinal microflora. In the presence of DSS the absorption of tartrazine is increased from 7 to 55 per cent, leading to a much higher blood and brain level than would ordinarily occur.

There is practically no information in the literature concerning the absorption of food additives and their distribution in tissues, including the brain. Rat pups can be treated with a substance called 6-hydroxydopamine and this tends to deplete brain dopamine, resulting in a syndrome which is similar to minimal brain dysfunction (MBD) in children. The activity in these so-called hyperactive rats was significantly greater than that found in control rats which had not been administered 6-hydroxydopamine. This hyperactivity was increased still further if the rats ingested food colourings in the order of 2mg/kg. The activity level of even normal pups fed food dyes was also increased. The performance in T-maze and shuttlebox is impaired in hyperactive rats and was not further affected by the addition of food colourings to the diet. However, escape latency in both T-maze and shuttlebox was impaired in normal rat pups following ingestion of food colouring mixtures. These findings demonstrate that food colourings may affect both activity level and cognitive function, at least in rodents, and raise the possibility that adverse effects may develop in normal as well as hyperactive children.

Dr. Robert Buckley from the Hayward Vesper Hospital in Hayward, California, points out the similarity in toxicity of an azoaniline sulphur antibiotic dye called Prontosil (see Figure 2.13) and the toxic responses that have occurred as a result of tartrazine (F, D, and C Yellow No. 5 ingestion). When the structure of tartrazine is analysed it is found to contain two molecules of sulphanilic acid. This is a precursor chemical used in the manufacture of sulphanilamide. Looking at the development of sulphanilamide as a drug reveals that it was once linked

Figure 2.13 Similarity in chemical structures (and toxicity) of the azo food dye tartrazine and the antibiotic Prontosil

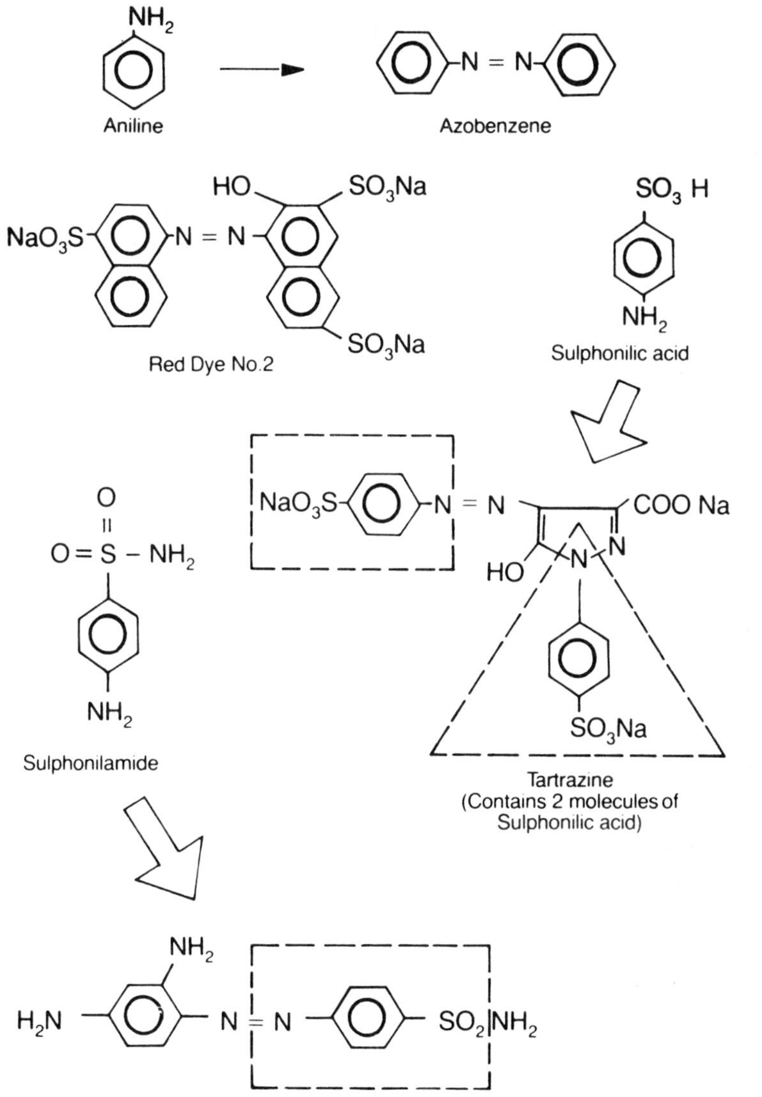

Prontosil
(Red dye and antibiotic – liberates sulphonilamide in the gut)

to a red dye marketed as the first truly important antibiotic drug, Prontosil.

Buckley points out that in the 1920s all the major chemical companies were looking for safe new chemicals that could destroy dangerous bacteria. The I.G. Farben Corporation in Germany found that sulphanilamide was just such a chemical. The problem was that Farben had developed and patented sulphanilamide many years previously when they were developing special textile dyes, and the patent had run out. If they had released the news about sulphanilamide being an effective antibiotic then the company would not have had sole rights, and any other company could have made it. So they then linked sulphanilamide to a red dye by an azo double bond, and the new chemical was not an adequate antibiotic until it was taken by mouth. This meant that the azo dye antibiotic would split in the stomach to release the antibiotic and the sulphanilamide that was released would be absorbed by the patient. The construction of this new chemical won a Nobel Prize for the maker. It also took other scientists a couple of years to discover that sulphanilamide was the active principal contained in Prontosil.

Tartrazine is a molecule that is very similar in structure to Prontosil. It is an azo dye with one sulphanilic acid molecule, linked to the larger chemical by an azo double bond which is also broken up when it is metabolised by intestinal bacteria. Both molecules of sulphanilic acid can be released and absorbed by the patient and are excreted in the urine. Buckley has proposed that some of the toxic qualities of sulphanilamide are shared by sulphanilic acid. This can account for the fact that tartrazine appears to be more likely to cause sensitivity reactions than other grass dyes. Even if a certain amount of the tartrazine is absorbed intact, there is at least good evidence that because of the metabolism by normal bacteria there will also be a fairly high quantity of sulphanilic acid absorbed.

Benjamin Urschoff from the Institute for Nutritional Studies in Culver City, California has shown that three food additives can be far more toxic when they are given together than when they are taken separately. When growing rats are placed on a low-fibre nutritious diet and given F, D and C Red No. 2 singularly, or the food sweetener Cyclamate, or the surface wetting agent Tween 60, there were no untoward reactions. However, when two of the chemicals were given together, many of the rats became sick and died, but when all three of the chemical substances were given simultaneously to the same group of growing rats, all of them died within two weeks. Urschoff further showed that when an apparently non-toxic quantity of cyclamate is given together with refined table sugar (sucrose), the cyclamate suddenly becomes toxic. So this information, arising from animal studies, suggests that there is a definite toxic interaction between different substances such as food dyes, sweeteners and surface wetting agents.

There is also an adverse interaction between various refined foods and some of these agents, in addition to the cumulative effect of ingesting food additives together. When it is considered that many hundreds, perhaps thousands, of these different food additives are consumed each day with varying diets and together with varying amounts of drugs, and perhaps antibiotics, it is no wonder that many people are complaining of adverse reactions from food additives.

One very interesting study carried out by James Swanson from The Research Institute Hospital for Sick Children, Toronto, Ontario, Canada, and Marcel Kinsbourne, Department of Psychology, University of Toronto, Ontario, Canada examined the influence of nine different food dyes in doses of 100–150mg on the performance of hyperactive children in a laboratory learning test. Forty children were given a diet free of artificial food dyes and other additives for five days. Twenty of these children had been classified as hyperactive by scores on the Connor's rating scale, and reported to have favourable reponses to stimulant medication. A diagnosis of hyperactivity had been rejected in the other twenty children. Oral challenges with large doses, i.e. 100–150mg of a blend of F, D and C approved dyes or placebo were administered on days four and five of the experiment. The performance of the hyperactive children on paired associate learning tests on the day they received the dye blend was impaired relative to the performance after they received the placebo, but the performance of the non-hyperactive group was not affected by the challenge with the food dye blend. The researchers note that 150mg challenge dose of food dyes is more than ten times the amount used in most previous studies. They report that elsewhere no significant dye-induced impairment in performance on their laboratory learning test occurred when 20mg of food dye blend (i.e. the Nutrition Foundation's underestimate of daily consumption) was given in a single dose.

When a blend of dyes is used, a high dose may be necessary to elicit a behavioural response in hyperactive children and this might be true for animals as well. It is therefore not surprising that experiments by other investigators have shown little or no effect when small amounts of individual azo dyes are given. In this study the toxic effects of small amounts of nine azo dyes was shown to be additive. Children received 90 per cent of the amount that the FDA had said was the maximum safe or non-toxic amount for use in one day. This study confirms Benjamin Urschoff's proposal that the stress responses of some of the food additives combine with each other.

Most of the findings indicate that the research, even though performed as double-blind controlled trials, has been inadequate. The amount of substances used in testing has been insufficient and many of the children suffering from behavioural disturbances frequently ingest huge amounts of foods containing multiple food additives as well as other chemicals. Toxicological programs used to examine new colouring agents and food additives are inadequate in that they do not examine the possible adverse behaviour effects of these.

3

Asthma, skin disorders and food additives

Each one of us is biochemically unique. Some may have a greater requirement for a certain micronutrient than others. Infants born with a genetically greater requirement for vitamin B6, for example, have convulsive seizures unless they are given extra quantities of the vitamin. Some people are born with a defect in amino acid metabolism such as those with phenylketonuria (PKU). These individuals cannot metabolise one of the protein amino acids called phenylalanine and have to go on a strict elimination diet.

When we have an important biological molecule or a whole physiological system either completely missing, working suboptimally or working incorrectly, we can often compensate in some way and still function relatively normally until some unforeseen stress suddenly arises placing an extra burden on the weakened area. This can happen in many ways. Patients contracting kidney disease cannot handle extra protein and are unable to eliminate even small levels of the toxic mineral, aluminium, which can quickly build up to cause neurological damage (encephalopathy). A malfunctioning liver with abnormal liver enzymes as a result of hepatitis, alcoholism or chronic drug intake can prevent a person from detoxifying drugs and other chemicals which subsequently leads to toxic accumulations in the body.

While most people do not have major genetic defects and can adequately cope with their environment, there is a small sub-

group of the population with genetic or environmentally induced susceptibilities who have a real problem in handling
specific chemicals ingested with food. Some of these chemicals
are food additives. Extensive toxicological screening of these
agents is still no guarantee for the person with specific chemical
handling defects. One of the best examples of this type of
chemical hypersensitivity is the adverse reactions of some to the
common food preservative, metabisulphite.

There have always been people who complain about restaurant food and it is not uncommon to read reports of people
suffering from food poisoning, but it's only in the last ten years
that reports have come through of people having to be
hospitalised due to ingesting food additives in restaurant food.
Ten years ago a middle-aged man with no history of allergies
suddenly found himself hospitalised after eating restaurant
food. The additive responsible in this case was sodium bisulphite, and further testing of the skin of this patient produced the
classic weal indicative of chemical sensitivity. A similar report
appeared in the *Journal of the American Medical Association* in 1982
of an asthmatic woman finding that she experienced recurrent
episodes of wheezing when she ate restaurant food, ending up
on many occasions in hospital. It was only after some of the
drugs that she was taking during hospitalisation produced
adverse reactions that the doctors found that the culprit was
bisulphite in both foods and drugs. There have now been seven
deaths reportedly due to sulphite hypersensitivity reactions in
the United States and it is thought that as many as 450,000 of
the nation's asthma sufferers may have such a sensitivity. A ten-
year-old girl in Salem went out to a restaurant with her family
and found that she began to suffer chest pains and shortness of
breath. She lost consciousness on the way to hospital and died
five days later; again bisulphite reaction was suspected. Oregon's
Health Division had planned to issue warnings about bisulphite
sensitivity, but when this particular case came up, it issued
emergency rules requiring restaurants to stop using sulphites or
to post warnings at restaurant entrances and on menus. The
Oregon Restaurant and Beverage Association which represents
about nine hundred of an estimated six thousand restaurants
prefers a ban to a warning. They believe that restaurant owners
are reluctant to start plastering their walls with different labels

and believe that health warnings should come from physicians. The Washington State Board of Health has recently banned the use of sulphites completely and it is thought that many other American states may follow suit.

Presently a variety of sulphiting agents including sulphur dioxide and some inorganic sulphites are being used as preservative substances. They prevent microbial spoilage and also act as antioxidants to prevent lettuces and other fruits and vegetables from going brown. After sulphite treatment vegetables maintain their fresh appearance even though they may be quite old and stale. This is particularly evident in restaurants that have salad bars. The popular use of these has made it a necessity to present vegetables fresh in appearance. Sulphites are also used to sanitise containers as selective inhibiters of undesirable organisms in the fermentation industries. It is thought that people attending restaurants may consume anywhere from 25– 100mg of metabisulphite in one meal. Since many bottles of wine contain up to 350ppm of sulphite, it is quite easy to see how a person may overload on sulphite after drinking half a bottle of wine (which could contain at least 125mg) as well as eating at the salad bar (what they consume could contain that much again).

Twenty per cent of sulphites in wines exist in the form of sulphur dioxide. Recommended levels of sulphur dioxide in dehydrated fruits and vegetables could start at very high levels, but over a period of time it is lost so that only 10 per cent of the original content used in the drying process of dried apricots, may remain if a long period of time goes by in storage. This could amount to 56mg of sulphur in an ounce of dried apricots. There are actually six sulphiting agents. These are sulphur dioxide, sodium sulphite, sodium bisulphite, potassium bisulphite, sodium metabisulphite and potassium metabisulphite. Up until now an unsuspecting public has been ingesting many foods containing one of these six sulphite substances. They are currently added to or sprayed on fresh fruit, vegetables, shellfish, prawns, chicken, bread, sweet pastries, crackers, fresh mushrooms, frozen pizzas, dehydrated potatoes, some prepared lemon juices, vinegar, sauerkraut, relish, olives, beer and wine, potato purée, fruit juice, soft drinks, cordial, cider, sausages, pickles especially pickled onions, cheese mixtures and pastes, dehydrated fruits and vegetables, French fried potatoes, commercially prepared fresh fruit salad and potato crisps, to name the major ones (see Figure 3.1).

In an acid solution many of the bisulphites are in equilibrium with sulphur dioxide so that in orange juice, which is acid, the equilibrium between sodium or potassium metabisul-

---

Figure 3.1   Foods containing metabisulphite

DRINKS

Commercial bottled drinks containing soft drinks (soda) or fruit juice
Cordials
Cider (with preservatives)
Beer
Champagne
Wines (sweet wines 35mg/glass, dry wines 10–15mg/glass)

FRUIT

Dried tree fruits such as apples, apricots, pears (not raisins, sultanas, currants or prunes)
Fruit bars
(Fresh fruit salad from commercial outlets may have metabisulphite added to help maintain fresh appearance)

VEGETABLES

Dried vegetables
Instant mashed potato
Pickled onions
Sauerkraut
Pickles
Commercially prepared (cut, dehydrated, peeled or chipped) potatoes
Some potato crisps and fresh mushrooms

MEAT/FISH/POULTRY

Brawn, chicken loaf, devon, frankfurters, sausages, sausage mince, uncooked fresh prawns (shrimp), shellfish

DAIRY PRODUCTS

Fruit yoghurt, cheese pastes

OTHERS

Dessert toppings, flavouring essences, jams, vinegar, vinegar-containing items (salad dressings, sauces, relish), olives, tomato purée, tomato paste, some breads, frozen pizzas, sweet pastries, some crackers and cookies; also used in the processing of gelatin, beet sugar, corn sweeteners and food starches

Table 3.1   Amount of sulphite (expressed as sulphur dioxide) in typical servings of selected foods

	Typical serving	Total sulphite (mg/serve)
Cheese paste	30g	5–101
Fruit, dehydrated*	30g	45–90
Fresh fruit salad* (commercially prepared)	250–500g	NA
Fruit juices, soft drinks (soda), cordials*	250g	15–25
Pickles (such as pickled onions)*	15–30g	10–25
Potatoes (french fries)*	150g	NA
Potato crisps*	25–100g	NA
Sausages (and sausage meat)*	110g	40–45
Vegetables (dehydrated)	50g	25–75
Wine/Cider*	100ml	15–30

Note: * Sulphite containing foods which commonly provoke asthma
NA: Analysis not available
Source: Allen, D.H., Nussen, S.V., Loblay, R. *et al.* Adverse reactions to foods. *The Medical Journal of Australia* (special supplement) 1 September: S41 (1984)

phite and sulphite tends to favour sulphite and the liberation of gaseous sulphur dioxide (see Figure 3.2). So in a solution the relationship between the total amount of sulphite and the amount of sulphur dioxide and bisulphite is dependent on the acidity of the solution. When the pH is above 4, i.e. only moderately acidic, there is very little sulphur dioxide or bisulphite in the solution. However, at a pH of 2, which is very similar to that of the stomach pH, there is approximately 25 per cent of total sulphite in the sulphur dioxide form, while another 25 per cent will be in the form of bisulphite. There is now accumulating evidence which suggests that when an acid solution containing bisulphite or sulphur dioxide is taken by asthmatics, an asthma attack can be promoted within minutes of ingestion in a certain proportion of subjects.

In the past, researchers have found that a significant broncho-constriction can occur in asthmatic subjects after they inhale a gaseous mixture of sulphur dioxide in a concentration of only 1ppm for several minutes and even with lower concentrations. If subjects are exercising at the time of inhalation they will get bronchoconstriction, so exercise plus inhalation of sulphur dioxide can induce bronchoconstriction and an asthma attack. Exercising asthmatics may suffer at a level of only 1ppm sulphur dioxide. This concentration is often exceeded in polluted

Figure 3.2   Sulphiting agents

There are 6 of these:
  sodium sulphite
  sodium bisulphite
  potassium bisulphite
  sodium metabisulphite
  potassium metabisulphite
  sulphur dioxide

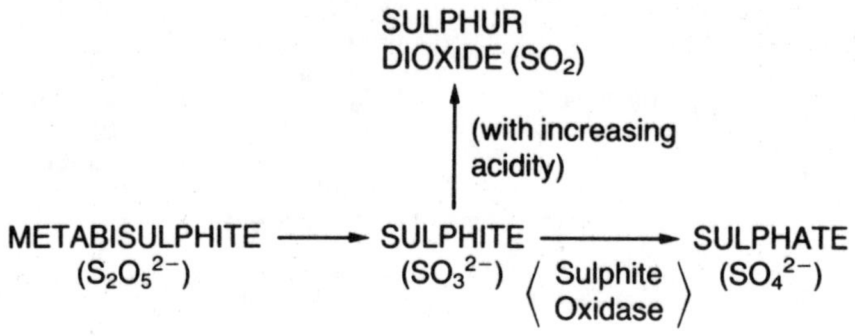

$$SULPHUR$$
$$DIOXIDE\ (SO_2)$$

(with increasing acidity)

$$METABISULPHITE \longrightarrow SULPHITE \longrightarrow SULPHATE$$
$$(S_2O_5{}^{2-}) \qquad\qquad (SO_3{}^{2-}) \left\langle \begin{array}{l} Sulphite \\ Oxidase \end{array} \right\rangle (SO_4{}^{2-})$$

In acid solutions such as citrus juices, a percentage of sulphite or metabisulphite is converted into sulphur dioxide.

After absorption of sulphites into the body they are rapidly metabolised to sulphate by the enzyme sulphite oxidase; this is malfunctional in individuals with sulphite sensitivity.

urban air and also in many industrial workplaces. Even normal individuals may develop bronchospasm at a sulphur dioxide level of 6ppm and in asthmatics who are not exercising, at a level of only 1ppm.

In industrial countries coal or oil fired electric power plants probably account for 75 per cent of sulphur dioxide emission. Sulphites are also found in a number of parenteral medications, as well as analgesics, anaesthetics, steroids and nebulised bronchodilators. It is always wise to check with the drug company to see if any of the drugs have sulphites in them. It is ironic that many of the drugs that are used to ease respiratory distress due to bronchospasm in asthmatics, may contain metabisulphite. These include Dexamethozone, Adrenaline, Bronchoepherin, Bronchosol, Isuprel, and Metaprel. Metacholpromide is commonly used to ease gastrointestinal distress in asthmatics and allergic individuals, and it also contains metabisulphite; there have been reports of life-threatening asthma episodes after administration of this drug.

A recent study at a children's hospital in Sydney showed that asthma in up to 65 per cent of patients, both children and adults, was provoked by ingestion of foods or beverages containing metabisulphite. Typical symptoms that patients experienced were a tightening in the throat soon after eating the food, followed by asthma, which could be quite severe. The attack usually lasted for thirty to forty minutes but could be terminated by the use of an inhaled bronchodilator.

The study examined twenty-nine children with chronic asthma. After a week on a strict elimination diet all twenty-nine were challenged with placebo in a single-blind fashion on three consecutive days in the pulmonary function laboratory, and then given metabisulphite in both capsule form and solution. Children with a positive response to metabisulphite were then prescribed a diet that excluded all foods containing it. After three months on restricted diets the children were reassessed to determine whether there had been any therapeutic improvement, and were challenged again with metabisulphite. They found that there was a 66 per cent incidence of positive challenge, i.e. nineteen of the children responded with a 20 per cent decrease in forced expiratory volume (FEV) in one second after they took the metabisulphite challenge solution, which had been acidified. They did not, however, react when metabisulphite was given in capsule form. After three months on the diet restricted in metabisulphites and sulphur dioxide, four of the nineteen children had objective signs of improvement which included a reduction in asthma medications and/or improvement in lung function. Unfortunately, compliance with the diet during the three-month period was very poor. It was concluded that long-term elimination of these substances from a child's diet is difficult and does not in general improve a chronic asthma condition.

The symptoms that the children experienced when they were first challenged with metabisulphite solutions included a burning sensation in the throat followed by a tight cough, an audible wheeze and signs of respiratory distress. This usually occurred within the first minute after ingestion and was associated with a decrease in peak expiratory flow rate (PEFR) of 39 per cent with a range of between 23–72 per cent decrease in mean PEFR. The mean decrease in forced expiratory volume (FEV) was 33 per

cent, with a range from 22 to 66 per cent. Eighty-four per cent
of the children (sixteen of nineteen) reacted within two minutes
with symptoms. For the remaining three children it took fifteen
minutes, and the mean duration of the reaction to metabisulphite was thirteen minutes, with subsequent spontaneous
recovery in seventeen.

Seven of the nineteen, i.e. 37 per cent, had a history of reactions to metabisulphite and this most commonly occurred to
pickled onions and commercially prepared orange juice. Four of
the children had a subjective improvement in their asthma
symptoms and two reported that they no longer required
regular doses of bronchodilator at night while on the two week
elimination diet. However, comparison of the daily symptoms
score and the PEFR rate showed no significant differences between week one and week two. After three months on the
metabisulphite restricted diet only one child had a dramatic
response, with improvement in pulmonary function, a decrease
in bronchodilator therapy and marked subjective improvement.
The metabisulphite-free diet did not involve radical changes in
food consumption and alternative foods and beverages not containing metabisulphite could be substituted with ease. It is
possible that the poor compliance with these special diets was
the reason for the lack of a more dramatic response in other
children when on a metabisulphite-free diet. It is noteworthy,
however, that none of the children's asthmatic conditions
worsened during the period that they were on the restricted
diet. Compliance was so bad, however, that it makes one think
that had the children persisted with the restricted diet the results
may have been much better.

At this stage it is very difficult to say that a metabisulphite-
free diet is *not* going to lead to a reduction in bronchospasms
and asthma attacks. It must be kept in mind, however, that
strict dietary avoidance has proved impractical, is associated
with poor compliance and, at least at this stage, did not appear
generally to result in improvement in asthma, either objectively
or subjectively.

The fact that asthmatics tend to react to the metabisulphite
acidified solution but not to capsules of metabisulphite swal-
lowed prompted some research by Dr. David Allen at the
Department of Thoracic Medicine, Royal North Shore Hospi-

tal in Sydney. Dr. Allen took three groups with ten subjects in each group, groups one and two being asthmatics. Group one asthmatic subjects were known to react to metabisulphite, and group two was found to be non-reactors to ingested metabisulphite. A third group consisted of non-asthmatic control subjects. All subjects were challenged with metabisulphite on separate days, with 50mg in citric acid and sulphur dioxide gas at increasing concentrations of 0.5, 1.5, 3 and 5ppm. The mean fall in peak expiratory flow rate after the ingestion of metabisulphite for group one was 35 per cent, for group two 6 per cent and for group three 5 per cent. The mean sulphur dioxide provocation concentration for group one was 1.19ppm while for group two it was double this, at 2.25ppm, while the control group was greater than 5ppm. Hence the metabisulphite-sensitive asthmatics demonstrated the greatest airways resistance at the lowest concentration of metabisulphite or sulphur dioxide.

Five of the metabisulphite-sensitive subjects were then challenged with metabisulphite solution by a mouthwash or a naso-gastric tube. While asthma was provoked in all five subjects by the mouthwash, it was not provoked when the metabisulphite was introduced directly into the stomach by tube. These results suggest that the metabisulphite-sensitive asthmatics are probably reacting to the release of sulphur dioxide when the metabisulphite hits stomach acid and is inhaled. It has been previously shown that a concentration of inhaled sulphur dioxide gas of less than 1ppm arising from the stomach is enough to provoke an asthma attack in susceptible asthmatics at rest. The fact that the introduction of metabisulphite solution into the stomach by naso-gastric tube failed to produce asthma indicated that gastrointestinal absorption was not an important provoker. Two mechanisms appear to be important. Firstly, there are special sulphite-sensitive receptors in the mouth that initiate an orobronchial reflex causing reflex spasm of the bronchial tubes. Alternatively, variable inhalation of sulphur dioxide gas, while mouthwashing or swallowing the metabisulphite solution, provoked bronchospasm, i.e. group one subjects continued to breathe while mouthwashing or swallowing while group two ones breathed less or not at all.

Dr. Allen has observed that an asthmatic is quite likely to get an attack after ingesting metabisulphite if after it reaches stomach acid and releases sulphur dioxide, the person burps. One burp could probably produce 3 or 4ppm which, when breathed in, is enough to elicit bronchospasm and perhaps an attack.

In 1974 the World Health Organization felt that an acceptable daily intake of sulphur dioxide per kilogram human body weight per day was between 0 and 0.7mg sulphur dioxide. It was thought that most mammalian tissue oxidises sulphur dioxide to sulphate as shown in Figure 3.2.

The system responsible for this conversion is located in most cells between the membranes of the microchondria, the power houses of the cells. The enzyme system, sulphite oxidase, has been shown to be a molybdenum dependent one, deficiencies of sulphite oxidase have been produced in animals by maintaining them on low molybdenum diets and treating them with a heavy metal such as tungsten, which is known to compete with molybdenum for use in living systems. It is interesting to speculate whether some of the heavy metal pollutants in the environment such as lead and mercury are also in some way competing with major enzyme systems such as sulphite oxidase. It was found that animals treated with tungsten or one of these heavy metals in this way were more susceptible to bisulphite toxicity. Furthermore the sulphite oxidase activity in rat liver is negligible at birth, but increases rapidly between five and eleven days after birth, and is very much impaired by the administration of tungsten for twenty days before the delivery of litters. This indicates that the effect on the foetus cannot be discounted if the mother is subjected to a large amount of heavy metal.

Sulphur dioxide has also been shown to react with a variety of biological molecules such as blood plasma proteins, probably by removing the disulphide bridges that form different layers of a protein molecule. This is very important if the bridge is the critical disulphide one such as occurs in the insulin molecule. It is thought by some that the marked alteration in carbohydrate metabolism that is observed after exposure to sulphite or sulphur dioxide is perhaps due to destruction of these sulphur bonds of biologically active substances such as insulin controlling the rate of entry of glucose into our cells. Glucose tolerance tests have indicated that disturbed carbohydrate metabolism

Figure 3.3

Power station pollution and asthma
The front page of the *Sydney Morning Herald* for 31 October 1985 carried a story on the association between respiratory complaints and pollution emanating from two power stations situated in a township a hundred kilometres north of Sydney. The report stated that 40 per cent of children attending the public school, which is situated between the two large power stations, suffered from some form of respiratory complaint. Three general practitioners working in the area have estimated that the incidence of asthma in children under twelve is 30 per cent — twice the national average. Non-smoking adults with recurrent bronchitis were also reported in greater number than normal. Recently the public school was forced to cancel its daily fifteen-minute recreational run because so many children were unable to participate as a result of asthma or other respiratory complaints. Most of the parents contacted said that their children had only contracted asthma after moving into the area. The fallout arising from the power stations and causing all the problems is thought to be sulphur dioxide gas.

occurs in rabbits which are exposed to 50–100ppm of sulphite or sulphur dioxide for two hours each day for up to six months.

Interference with bonds may also affect the structural integrity of immunoglobulins and contribute in part to the observed adverse effects of sulphur dioxide on antibody response. Reduced antibody formation was exhibited by rabbits exposed for eighty days, nine and a half hours a day, to sulphur dioxide in air at a concentration of 36mg/cubic metre. Occupational safety and health administration in the United States allows workers to be exposed to 10mg/cubic metre as a time-weighted average, very close to 36mg/cubic metre over eighty days.

Sulphur dioxide may also be involved with reactions with our genetic material DNA and RNA. It has been shown that sulphur dioxide reacts with some of the nucleotides, cytosine and urocil, and it has been cited as the basis of mutogenic effects in microorganisms. It also inhibits double helix formation and modifies template activity in DNA. It interferes with transcription and inactivates RNA in coding for protein synthesis in model systems. The possibility of similar responses in humans either at the tissue level or in relation to organisms in the gastrointestinal tract which contribute towards optimal digestion appears worthy of consideration. It is now well known that sulphur dioxide will inactivate dietary thiamine (vitamin B1) but there is growing information that it also interacts with folic acid and some of the flavines (riboflavin, vitamin B2) and flavo-enzymes, and also vitamin K. Dr. K. Pfeiffer of Princeton Brain BioCentre believes that a possible explanation for sulphite sensitivity might be the widespread molybdenum deficiency which he finds in a majority of his patients. Many had no de-tectable blood molybdenum and most had levels below 5ppb (normal levels range from 10–100ppb). This may prove to be an important finding as molybdenum is the trace element that is necessary to activate sulphite oxidase which, as has been noted, detoxifies sulphite to harmless sulphate. It is quite possible in countries such as Australia and New Zealand, where there is a molybdenum deficiency in the soils, that the accumulation of toxic sulphite may in fact be due to a deficiency of molybdenum and hence a deficiency in some individuals of sulphite oxidase. Foods high in molydenum are legumes such as soy beans and lentils. Extra supplementation may be quite prudent for sulphite-sensitive individuals or for anyone who is exposed to undue amounts of sulphite-containing foods, drugs, heavy metals, or smog. It might also be advantageous for such indi-viduals to take vitamin C and thiamine because both of these are depleted by excessive exposure to metabisulphites and sulphur dioxides. Pfeiffer also claims that pantothenic acid has been shown to foster significant protection against sulphur dioxide poisoning. Sulphites are now considered to be the hidden trigger in up to 10 per cent of asthmatics, i.e. nearly one million Americans. While sulphite sensitivity occurs mainly in this group, the FDA states that 30 per cent of reported cases occur in non-asthmatics with no known allergies.

Aspirin also appears to play a role in some children's chronic asthma. In the same study where chronic asthmatic children were challenged with metabisulphite, 66 per cent of them were found to have a decrease in forced expiratory volume, and 21 per cent also found to react adversely to aspirin. These six of twenty-nine children reacting to aspirin after oral challenge also showed up positive in reaction to skin testing and all reacted to 150mg of aspirin with a greater than 20 per cent decrease in both peak expiratory flow rate and forced expiratory volume in one second. The mean decrease in PEFR was 37 per cent, with a

Figure 3.4

Metabisulphite toxicity and vitamin B12
A 37-year-old man with allergic reactions to metabisulphite suffered for 15 years from symptoms of hepatotoxicity, ulcerative colitis, and skin disorders including itching and redness. The patient was placed on a metabisulphite-free diet and all symptoms improved. When metabisulphite was added to the diet, symptoms returned. However, when 3mg vitamin B12 was administered concurrently with the metabisulphite, toxicity symptoms were prevented. The researchers concluded that vitamin B12 might be an effective agent in the prevention of metabisulphite toxicity. Flaherty M., Stormont J., Condemi J. Metabisulphite (MBS) — associated hepatoxicity and protection by cobalamines (B12) J. Allerg. Cl. 75, 198 (1985)

range from 28–73 per cent, while the decrease in forced expiratory volume was 33.8 per cent, with a range of from 21–50 per cent. All had obvious clinical response with signs of respiratory distress and generalised bronchi on osculation of the chest and were advised to avoid the aspirin-containing medications. Five of the six were also given advice, including written information, regarding dietary avoidance of natural salicylates. Compliance was very poor and was continued on an average for only three weeks. Two other reports have shown that the incidence of aspirin sensitivity in asthmatic children was about 13 and 28 percent respectively.

Another study reported by Tarlow and Broler in 1982 found that after a month on an avoidance diet not only was there no improvement, but the majority of patients experienced a worsening of asthmatic symptoms and an increase in medication was required. Because aspirin-sensitive patients may become refractory to the adverse effects of it by its daily ingestion, it is possible that an avoidance diet could render them more sensitive to even small amounts of accidentally ingested aspirin and naturally occurring salicylates in foods, resulting in a deterioration of their asthmatic condition. For this reason it is suggested that children and adults with aspirin hypersensitivity must avoid medicinal aspirin. But avoidance of naturally occurring salicylates in foods is not only difficult and does not alter a child's asthma, but could potentially make him or her more sensitive to aspirin and salicylates in general. So while it is not considered appropriate to place a child on a salicylate-free diet, it probably is appropriate to place him or her on a diet low in salicylate.

Animal experiments have shown that aspirin can greatly increase the permeability of the intestinal tract to foreign proteins and that this effect is delayed by about thirty minutes. So if aspirin is taken together with a potential food allergen, the situation could become life-threatening. A recent report illustrates this point well. A fourteen-year-old boy who had suffered from eczema, asthma and hayfever since his early childhood had eaten foods containing peanuts on several occasions since the age of two and found adverse reactions within seconds. This was characterised by tingling and dryness of the lips and mouth, followed by swelling of the lips and face, with a sensation of choking in the throat. Usually these manifestations passed within about five minutes. Though he had taken aspirin on several previous occasions with no ill-effects, on the day that he was admitted to hospital he had a mild headache and had taken two 300mg tablets. Five minutes after he had taken the aspirin he had eaten a piece of cake containing peanuts. While he suffered his usual reaction to peanuts, within five minutes he was perfectly well again. However, thirty minutes after eating the cake he began to feel unwell, with generalised pruritis (severe itching), a choking sensation and extreme shortness of breath. He then collapsed. On admission to hospital he was unconscious, deeply cyanosed (bluish-coloured skin due to lack of oxygen) and covered with an urticarial rash. He had a rapid pulse rate, his blood pressure was 120/80, breath sounds were quiet and there was little wheeze. Electrocardiography showed atrial ectopic (extra) beats with periods of sinus arrest (initiating impulses for the heart beat stop). He had to be given intravenous adrenaline, sodium bicarbonate, aminophyllin, hydrocortisone and chlorpheniramine, after which he made a dramatic recovery: within ten minutes he was conscious with a mild wheeze. Forty-five minutes after admission he was completely free from symptoms and remained well thereafter.

Other studies have also shown that twenty to thirty minutes

after the introduction of aspirin into the stomach the absorption of substances with large molecular weights of up to 7,000 was greatly increased. The change in permeability permits the development of anaphylaxis to molecules normally too large to cross the gastric mucosa. Anaphylaxis is delayed while the changes induced by aspirin take place. It is thought that aspirin increases the antigen (foreign protein) uptake by perhaps blocking the pro-inflammatory prostaglandin E_2 (a substance which promotes inflammation), hence activating damaging leukotriene (substances made from fats that are involved in inflammatory processes) pathways. The fact that the ingestion of aspirin together with potential food allergens may bring on unexpectedly severe and life-threatening reactions suggests that patients who suffer even mild immediate hypersensitivity reactions to foods should be warned that they could suffer a severe reaction if they take the offending allergen together with aspirin.

Between 10–20 per cent of asthmatic children and adults have some sort of adverse reaction to aspirin if it's taken on an empty stomach; an attack, which could be life-threatening will commence twenty to forty minutes later. Compounds contain-

Figure 3.5

Pharmaceutical preparations containing aspirin or salicylate available in Australia		
Alka-Seltzer	Codis	Percodan
Ancosal	Codox	Phumax
Asco(tin)	Codral blue label	Rhusal
Aspalgin	Codral forte	Salamide
Aspirin BP	Decrin	Salicylamide
Aspro Clear	Disprin	Sodium salicylate
Aspro regular	Dolobid	Solcode
Bayer Aspirin	Doloxene Co	Solprin
Benoral	Ecotrin	Solusal
Bex powders	Elsprin	Solusal-Co
Bex tablets	Ensalate	SRA
Bi-prin	Equagesic	Veganin
Bufferin 500	Florinal	Vincents powers
Code-Co	Hycodin	Vincents tablets
Codiphen	Morphalgin	Winsprin
Codiphen forte	Palaprin forte	

Figure 3.6

Non-steroidal anti-inflammatory drugs
Sodium salicylate (ensalate)
Phenylbutazone (Butazolidin, Butalgin, BTZ)
Oxyphenbutazone (Tanderil)
Indomethacin (Indocid, Rheumacin)
Sulindac (Clinoril)
Mefenamic acid (Ponstan)
Flufenamic acid (Arlef)
Tolmetin (Tolectin)
Naproxen (Naprosyn)
Ibuprofen (Orudis)
Ketoprofen (Orudis)
Deflunisal (Dolobid)
Fenoprofen (Fenopron)
Zomepirac

ing aspirin in Australia are listed in Figure 3.5. It should also be noted that patients insensitive to aspirin usually react to other non-steroidal anti-inflammatory agents (see Figure 3.6). Care should always be taken in administering any form of analgesic agent to a patient who has a severe reaction to an anti-inflammatory drug: the first dose should be given under hospital care as a challenge.

Dr. David Allen from the Royal North Shore Hospital, Sydney, has noted that aspirin sensitivity treatment is either avoidance or desensitisation. Other workers have shown that when patients are challenged with aspirin and then maintained on 650mg four times a day they become tolerant and it does not provoke asthma, but the best treatment is merely avoidance of the aspirin. The yellow food dye, tartrazine, and other similar dyes have also been shown to provoke asthma. Frequently there is a cross-reactivity and patients sensitive to tartrazine are also sensitive to aspirin. Studies carried out at the Royal North Shore Hospital have indicated that up to 14 per cent of asthmatic patients are sensitive to tartrazine and should avoid all food containing it.

Research over the last few years has now also implicated many chemicals in provoking not only acute severe asthma but also urticaria and angioedema. Urticaria is described as discreet erythematis, oedematous itchy skin eruptions which usually last only a few hours at the same site. They can be localised or distributed over large areas of the body. While angioedema is a non-itchy swelling occurring under the skin, and also the mucous membranes of the face, eyelids, lips, tongue, hands and feet. Urticaria and angioedema are commonly produced by allergenic foods or chemicals and occur together in about 50 per cent of patients. Researchers from the Department of Clinical Immunology at Flinders Medical Centre in Bedford Park, South Australia have found about 34 per cent of chronic urticaria and angioedema sufferers with drug and diet related factors.

Intolerance to drugs and specific dietary factors are most important. There is strong evidence implicating penicillin, which after therapeutic administration to domestic animals, sometimes ends up in dairy products. Other drugs commonly involved are aspirin and sulphonamides, natural salicylates, and azo dyes, including tartrazine. Benzoates and related chemicals can also cause precipitation, perpetuation or exacerbation of chronic urticaria and angioedema. Substances such as flavouring agents, non-azo dyes, colouring agents and antioxidants are also implicated. (Salicylates occur naturally in many fruits, fruit juices, wines and some vegetables, and are frequently used in non-proprietary medications, perfumes and toothpaste.)

Patients presenting to the Flinders Medical Centre with persistent troublesome urticaria with no obvious cause are placed on a rigid diet excluding all forms of natural salicylates, colouring agents and preservatives. Patients whose urticaria subsides following the institution of this diet or who have infrequent urticaria are then challenged blind while withdrawn from all medication with capsules containing graded doses of aspirin benzoates, metabisulphite, tartrazine, penicillin and brewers yeast. Patients are also advised to avoid alcohol, aspirin, heat, exertion, and emotional stress, because all of these lower their threshold to urticaria. A similar procedure is followed at the Royal Prince Alfred Hospital Allergy Clinic in Sydney. Following confirmation of the diagnosis of chronic idiopathic urticaria and/or angioedema, patients are placed on a diet eliminating most food additives and other foods containing possible offending chemicals that may be naturally occurring. This elimination diet consists mainly of lamb, beef, chicken, turkey, veal potatoes, lettuce, parsley, pears, unpreserved bread, rice, plain flour, coffee, mineral water, milk, eggs, safflower and sunflower oils, sugar and golden syrup. After being maintained on this diet test substances are placed in capsules in clear gelatine and challenges are administered second daily in a random order. Test substances include aspirin, sodium benzoate, 4–hydroxy-benzoic acid, sodium metabisulphite, tartrazine, brewers yeast, starch, ascorbic acid, sodium nitrite, sodium nitrate, BHA, BHT, tyramine, phenylethylamine, MSG, gluten, lactose and sucrose (see Figure 3.7). A positive result is recorded if urti-

Figure 3.7   Challenges used for patients with urticaria and/or angioedema at Royal Prince Alfred Hospital, Sydney

Challenge compounds	Dose
Group 1 *	
Acetylsalicylic acid[†]	300 mg
Sodium Benzoate	500 mg ⎫
4-OH-benzoic acid	200 mg ⎬
Sodium metabisulphite[†]	500 mg ⎭
Tartrazine	30 mg
Brewers yeast	600 mg
Starch (placebo)	2 × 600 mg
Group 2	
Acetylsalicylic acid[†]	2 × 600 mg
Sorbic acid	200 mg
Sodium nitrite	100 mg ⎫
Sodium nitrate	100 mg ⎭
BHA (antioxidant)	50 mg ⎫
BHT (antioxidant)	50 mg ⎭
Tyramine	140 mg
Phenylethylamine	4 mg
MSG	2 × 2.8 g
Gluten	1.5 g
Lactose	700 mg
Sucrose (placebo)	2 × 700 mg

Notes: Brackets indicate challenge compounds that are taken together
          * Group 1 challenges are used for patients with urticaria alone; if patients have experienced systemic symptoms, both challenge groups are administered.
          † In asthmatic patients these compounds should only be taken under medical supervision. One quarter of the dose is taken every hour, provided there is no reaction. Patients should be kept under observation for at least 2 hours after the last dose
Source: Allen DH, Van Nunen S, Loblay R. *et al* Adverse reations to foods. *The Medical Journal of Australia* (special supplement) 1 September: S42 (1984)

caria and/or angioedema appears within twenty-four to forty-eight hours of administration of the test substances. If a positive result occurs, then further challenge is delayed for at least another forty-eight hours after lesions have subsided.

Approximately 90 per cent of patients with urticaria and angioedema have lesions appearing following one or more of the challenges. The most frequent reactions occur to tartrazine, sodium benzoate, benzoic acid, brewers yeast, aspirin, sodium salicylate, and sodium metabisulphite. Recurrent mouth ulcers, though infrequent, are characteristically found in salicylate-sensitive patients. In one group of seventy-six patients with chronic idiopathic urticaria referred to the Allergy Clinic at Royal Prince Alfred Hospital, seven refused the diet outright and four were lost to follow-up after challenge. One month after beginning the strict exclusion diet 65 per cent of the patients were in complete remission. By three months, 75 per cent were in remission. At challenge, 54 per cent of the patients reacted to salicylates, 34 per cent to benzoates or benzoic acid, 26 per cent to tartrazine, 12 per cent to yeast and 18 per cent to penicillin.

Twelve of the patients agreed to rechallenge after remaining on the diet for twelve months. Each was in complete remission. One patient failed to respond to the initial challenge and also gave no response at twelve months. Of four who initially responded to benzoate, three remained positive at twelve months. Of seven who responded initially to salicylates, five remained positive at twelve months. Of those initially reacting to tartrazine (three), penicillin (two) and yeast (one), all were negative to rechallenge with these substances. One patient who initially reacted to benzoate alone, reacted to benzoate *and* salicylate on rechallenge. Many patients noted that when they failed to maintain their diet their symptoms of urticaria returned. While some were successfully able to return to their previous food intake, 73 per cent of those retested after twelve months retained positive responses to challenge.

Foods allowed on this elimination diet included lamb, chicken, beef, veal and turkey (note that corned beef was not allowed); vegetables, including lettuce, carrot and parsley; fruit, including pears, fresh and canned; cereals, Mazo; biscuits, plain flour, semolina, rice, vermicelli, rice, Rice Bubbles, San Remo spaghetti and Carr's water biscuits. Fats included oils such as safflower and sunflower; sugars included cane sugar and golden syrup and honey; miscellaneous, malt, vinegar, salt, pepper and gelatin; beverages, coffee, pear nectar, homemade soups using the above ingredients and homemade desserts also using them.

The fact that urticaria could be induced by preservatives and dye additives in foods and drugs was known as far back as 1973. Then, workers at the Department of Dermatology at Uppsala University Hospital in Sweden worked with fifty-two patients with recurrent urticaria and angioedema, and with thirty-three controls. Each group was provoked with five different food dyes, including tartrazine, sunset yellow, new coccine, patent blue 5 and amaranth, with the preservative, sodium benzoate and 4-hydroxy-benzoic acid, as well as aspirin, sulphanilic acid and a placebo. The reaction was judged as positive in thirty-nine patients, who developed urticaria within fourteen hours. Of these, thirty-five reacted to aspirin, twenty-seven to benzoic acid compounds and twenty-seven to azo dyes. Four patients who did not have urticaria after aspirin reacted with urticaria after benzoic acid compounds, and three of them after azo dyes. None had any urticarial reaction to sulphanilic acid, patent blue (which is a non-azo dye) or the placebo. It was also found that in aspirin-sensitive patients, seven out of ten with recurrent urticaria and/or asthma reacted also to tartrazine.

A study published in the *British Journal of Dermatology* in 1976 by Robert Warren and Ruth Smith reported that out of a total number of a hundred and eleven patients, forty-five reacted to aspirin, twelve to sodium benzoate, five to 4-hydroxybenzoic acid, fourteen to tartrazine, fifteen to brewers yeast or Candida, and seventeen to penicillin. Some patients showed an exacerbation with two or more substances. This occurred particularly with aspirin and penicillin in twelve patients; with aspirin and tartrazine in eleven; and with aspirin and sodium benzoate in eight. More recently, Lenhard Julan from the Department of Dermatology University Hospital, Uppsala, Sweden, reported a clinical investigation involving three hundred and thirty patients with recurrent urticaria. Over one third of the patients had a history of allergies and just under one third had side effects from drugs, the commonest offenders being penicillin, aspirin, and sulphonamides. A similar proportion felt that their urticaria was exacerbated by food and fruits, particularly vegetables and nuts. For 20 per cent, heat and exercise were also factors. Severe depressions and psychiatric disorders affected 16 per cent. The researcher performed provocative tests with various food additives such as azo dyes, benzoates, BHA, BHT, ascorbic acid, quinoline yellow, carotene, canthaxanthine, orange dye annato and sodium nitrate. These provocative tests were performed on in-patients who had been free of urticaria and who had been stabilised on a salicylate and azo dye-free diet for four or five days. No antihistamines were given during the test period. One third of the subjects had a positive reaction to the food additives, one third showed negative reactions, and in the rest one or several tests were questionable. Twenty-two per cent of the patients reacted to aspirin, and between 10 and 20 per cent to azo dyes, benzoates, annato, beta carotene, BHA, BHT, quinoline yellow, canthaxanthine and yeast. Between 5 and 10 per cent reacted to lactose, sodium glutamate, sodium nitrite and ascorbic acid. Fifty-six patients were unable to tolerate soft drinks, fruit juices, wine, beer, alcoholic drinks or coffee; 38 per cent could not handle penicillin, 33 per cent aspirin, 21 per cent sulphonamides and between 4 and 10 per cent antihistamines, iron, iodide, indomethacin and tetracycline. Foods provoking urticaria were fruits, vegetables, nuts, fish, shellfish, spices, vanilla, eggs, milk products, cheese, bread, and fried foods, but particularly, fruit, fish, vegetables and nuts. About 10 per cent of the patients found that their urticaria got worse after exercise, sweating, heat, stress or nervousness.

Another provoker of a wide range of adverse effects in some individuals is the flavour enhancer, monosodium glutamate, commonly known as MSG. This substance is actually the sodium salt of the non-essential amino acid, glutamic acid, which occurs widely in all animal and vegetable proteins. In the past it has been used to enhance memory and intelligence, to help detoxify the ammonia which builds up in the body after hepatic coma and as an ingredient in the amino acid mixtures used for parenteral feedings. Until recently it has been considered a relatively safe food additive, as it is a normal constituent of our body, but now people are starting to view it with increasing suspicion.

Several animal studies have demonstrated that glutamic acid may produce brain lesions, particularly in newborn animals. This issue originated from the observation that high doses of glutamic acid produced lesions of the retina, destruction of neurones in the hypothalamus (a part of the brain) of newborn animals and neuro-endocrine disturbances. In 1969, Olny reported that infant mice between two and nine days of age injected subcutaneously with up to 4g of monosodium glutamate per kilogram and killed a few hours afterwards developed a selective lesion of the hypothalamus. There is an area of the hypothalamus rich in special cells thought to be dopaminergic and after administration of toxic doses of MSG about 80 per cent of the cells are destroyed. Acute neurotoxicity of MSG can also be induced in the rat, though neonatal rats are considerably less sensitive than mice to the neurotoxic effects of MSG. Lesions also occur when high doses of MSG are given subcutaneously or orally to guinea pigs and also to chickens, rabbits, and hamsters. The neurotoxic effects of MSG in monkeys is controversial. Olny and Sharp have reported that premature monkeys injected subcutaneously with high doses of MSG developed lesions in one area of the brain called the infundibular nucleus. Subsequently the same authors confirmed those findings in two other monkeys given MSG subcutaneously, and in three seven day old monkeys given MSG orally (1, 2 or 4g per kilogram). Finally, a pregnant monkey was injected intravenously with 2g/kg of MSG and the foetus delivered by Caesarian section showed typical lesions of the hypothalamus.

However, other studies of fifty-nine infant monkeys and six foetuses dosed with MSG *in utero* did not confirm the results of Olny and Sharp. Reynolds carefully tried to confirm the reproduction of hypothalamic lesions by MSG. In some experiments, plasma levels of MSG in the monkey foetus were elevated 400 times above basal values but still no lesions could be detected. It is possible that MSG may be neurotoxic only when other conditions occur simultaneously, as was probably the case in Olny's experiments, such as dehydration and poor conditions. Recent work indicates that MSG sensitivity may be particularly prevalent in animals or humans with vitamin B6 deficiency. It is also important to understand the difference between an irritative and a destructive lesion. Damage or induced neural malfunction doesn't necessitate morphological changes. Very few studies have shown that MSG passes through the placental barrier to the foetus, though one has found that very large doses of MSG injected subcutaneously in the late stages of pregnancy could induce typical hypothalamic lesions in the foetus. The dose of MSG must be very large because the operation of the highly effective placental barrier prevents the entry of glutamate into the foetus. It is known, however, that administration of relatively large doses of MSG to women does not affect the level of glutamic acid in their milk. In respect of the hypothalamic lesions it is interesting to note that the blood-brain barrier is represented by the fusion through tight junctions of brain capillary endothelial cells which convert the brain capillary wall into an epithelial barrier. This can be overcome only by two mechanisms, passive diffusion for fat-soluble compounds or carrier-mediated transport for water-soluble ones. Even a very large increase in plasma glutamic acid does not result in a change in the brain glutamic acid level. However, the fact that glutamic acid given even at high dose levels fails to induce changes in the whole brain glutamic acid level does not mean that certain areas of the brain are not permeable to its circulation. It appears that the hypothalamic area represents a special part of the brain in terms of the blood-brain barrier, and capillaries here have large porous areas instead of tight junctions. It is therefore possible that MSG diffuses from the extracellular space of this region to the sensitive areas of the brain.

While most research work evaluating the neurotoxic effects of glutamic acid or sodium glutamate has come to the conclusion that the risk of MSG neurotoxicity for man must be very low indeed, recent research carried out in Australia at Monash University's Pharmacology Department by Dr. Leslie Rogers indicates that glutamate may be able to pass through the blood-brain barrier of humans and that if MSG goes through to the brain it can affect young children more than adults because their blood-brain barriers are usually not strong enough. Children may thus be affected by MSG entering the brain and this may alter their learning ability and may even be the cause of several visual and behavioural problems. Rogers' research showed that chickens became retarded after being fed the equivalent of a normal daily dietary dose of MSG. Dr. Rogers believes that the blood-brain barrier does not develop to any extent in the foetus and perhaps even with the birth of the child. She says that one of the most dangerous times for consuming MSG is during pregnancy because glutamate may be able to get through the placenta to the foetus, and if the blood-brain barrier isn't formed in the foetus it could go on to the brain.

There is good evidence that MSG could be getting into the brain in some adults who suffer from Chinese Restaurant Syndrome, as well as children. Dr. Rogers suspects that the brain is involved because some of the symptoms include visual problems such as seeing flashing lights and hallucinating. It will be remembered that this syndrome is characterised by symptoms which include sensations of warmth in the face, a burning sensation in the skin, sweating, nausea and vomiting, and that it can also mimic myocardial infarction with stiffness, weakness in the limbs, tingling or pain in the chest radiating to both arms and back. Further symptoms may include palpitations, pressure headache, light-headedness, heartburn or gastric discomfort. The syndrome can occur very suddenly, within a few hours of ingesting MSG, or it can be delayed and occur six to twelve hours after ingestion. There have also been many cases recorded of upper respiratory distress and asthma.

Over a three year period thirty-two patients have been challenged with MSG at Royal North Shore Hospital and a number of these has experienced severe asthma. Twelve of the patients who reacted fell into two distinct groups. The first group who developed asthma did so with the additional symptoms of Chinese Restaurant Syndrome in one to two hours after the ingestion of MSG, while the second group didn't develop either symptoms or asthma until six to twelve hours after ingestion. The reaction to MSG was found to be dose dependent, and because it may be delayed by up to twelve hours, recognition is difficult for both patient and doctor. Because it is dose dependent it is most necessary for patients to gain an accurate estimate of how much MSG is in the foods that they are eating. In potentially sensitive individuals a dose of 0.5g is enough to elicit a response, and most patients react to

1.5–2g; some Chinese meals may contain 5–10g of MSG. In these cases it is likely to provoke severe asthma, so the amount is important. At this stage it is not known whether or not continued low or moderate intakes of MSG provoke asthma.

There is some evidence that the side-effect induced by MSG is produced only when there is a borderline deficiency of vitamin B6. A recent researcher took blood samples from a hundred and fifty-eight students who had not been taking any vitamin supplement. The red blood cells taken from them demonstrated that the vitamin B6-dependent enzyme glutamate oxalacetate transaminase was about 29 per cent less active than it could have been when excess pyridoxal 5-phosphate was added to the blood. Of these students, twenty-seven were chosen at random, and after fasting, each of the subjects was challenged in sequence with either a large dose of MSG (125mg/kg) or a placebo, in double-blind tests. Twelve of the twenty-seven showed characteristic symptoms of Chinese Restaurant Syndrome; the other fifteen did not. The twelve students who showed a symptomatic response were then told to take 50mg of pyridoxine a day, or a matching placebo for twelve weeks; they were then rechallenged with MSG. Eight of the nine subjects who proved on decoding to have received pyridoxine showed no response to the MSG, while all three students who had unknowingly received a placebo instead of vitamin B6 were still reacting adversely. This goes to show that under double-blind conditions adverse symptoms associated with MSG consumption can be ameliorated in a great majority of cases when vitamin B6 is taken with MSG.

It is also interesting to note that the activities of intestinal vitamin B6-dependent transaminase which utilises glutamic acid are lower in the neonate than in post-weanling rats, which may indicate that the newborn infant has a greater need for vitamin B6 as far as the metabolism of glutamic acid goes. MSG has been banned in Australia by the National Health and Medical Research Council for use in baby foods but the additive is still used widely in many other commercial food preparations that the baby may ingest.

Glutamate is usually found bound up in protein, and as one of the twenty-three odd naturally occurring amino acids it is

quite plentiful, constituting about 20 per cent of our daily
dietary protein. When in its bound form or in pieces of digested
protein called peptides it apparently does not have the same
adverse effects on susceptible people. It is only when it is in its
free form as glutamic acid or its sodium salt, sodium mono-
glutamate that adverse reactions arise. However, during food
processing there are various techniques such as boiling or
fermentation that can lead to the release of free glutamate. In
this way it can become freed from its bound form and with
these foods there is also the possibility of an adverse reaction to
free glutamate. As a result, MSG, the sodium salt of glutamic
acid can become elevated in the blood of people eating these
types of foods. In most Sydney supermarkets more than half
the tinned foods containing meat and vegetables: casseroles,
pastas, beef curries and Chinese food preparations, contain
MSG. As a result many children who have been weaned onto
solids may end up consuming large quantities of the additive.
The fact that Dr. Rogers found that chickens given MSG were
much slower to learn than chickens on a glutamate-free diet,
has some implications for children or infants ingesting large
amounts of glutamate. Clinical studies have linked MSG with
shudder attacks in children, and also in depression, hyperactivity and a depersonalisation and panic syndrome. Vicky
Riperre from the Institute of Psychiatry in London claims that
while unsystematic and anecdotal, these reports suggest that for
a minority of individuals MSG may be psychotoxic. Clearly the

Figure 3.8

Risk of methanol toxicity from artificial sweetener

A recent article has warned that Aspartame, an artificial sweetener for
diet sodas and soft drinks, may release toxic levels of methanol into
the bloodstream.

Aspartame (L-aspartyl-L-phenylalanine methyl ester) is said to
release methanol into the bloodstream through the small intenstine at
the rate of one molecule of methanol for each one of Aspartame.
Consumption of 1 litre of an Aspartame sweetened beverage may
result in ingestion of over 50mg of methanol.

(Monte W.C. Aspartame: methanol and the public health.
J. Applied Nutr. 36(1): 42–54 (1984))

wealth of existing evidence warrants further and more systematic investigation.

Special diets

The following two diet plans are examples of special food combinations that can be put together to remove or minimise the total quantity of food additives and naturally occurring reactive chemical agents. A low chemical-reactant diet (Grade 1) is a strict chemical free 'elimination diet' (which must be professionally supervised), while the Grade 2 plan is an example of a nutritionally safer and more balanced low-chemical diet.

The strict Low Chemical-Reactant Diet (Grade 1) is free from the following substances:

1. Cow's milk products (milk, cheese, butter, yoghurt, cream etc.)
2. Foods containing gluten (wheat, oats, rye, barley)
3. Yeasts and moulds
4. Salicylates
5. Benzoates (and other added preservatives); metabisulphites (sulphur dioxide); nitrites, etc.
6. Colouring agents such as tartrazine and other azo dyes, Erythrosine
7. Flavour enhancers such as MSG
8. Biologically active amines (histamine, serotonin, tyramine, phenylethylamine, theobromine, caffeine (and other xanthines)

After following this diet for one to six weeks, adverse reactions arising as a result of food chemical reactants should slowly subside. When all symptoms have disappeared each of the omitted potential chemical reactants should be introduced in small quantities, one at a time, every few days and possible adverse reactions noted so that specific substances can be avoided in future. It is not uncommon to find that some chemicals previously causing adverse reactions no longer do so after several months of controlled elimination dieting.

The more moderate Low Chemical-Reactant Diet (Grade 2) is still free from the major food additives, but it allows selected gluten and cow's milk products, with a wide variety of *low* salicylate fruits and vegetables. A *low* background level of yeasts, moulds and biologically active amines is present, but the overall reactant–chemical load is still very low.

This diet has a better nutritional balance than the Grade 1 diet (with the major food groups contributing the required daily macro and micronutrients). This is the recommended diet and should be followed for about three months before starting to

Figure 3.9   Low chemical-reactant diet (Grade 1)
(Strict — to be carried out in consultation with doctor, dietitian or nutritionist)

Foods permitted		Foods disallowed
Meat and Eggs	Beef, chicken flesh, lamb, turkey, veal, homemade hamburger mince, eggs	Bacon, pork, ham, organ meats, sausages, fish and seafood, overcooked meat, corned beef, canned meats, beef and chicken fat
Dairy Products and Oils	Cold pressed safflower and sunflower oils (free from any additives whatsoever)	Cooking oils (with added antioxidants), margarines, butter, cheese, yoghurt, powdered milk
Vegetables	Peeled potato, fresh parsley, lettuce	All other vegetables and commercial potato products such as crisps and chips
Nuts	Cashews	Peanuts, almonds
Fruit	Pears (peeled or canned in syrup not nectar or juice), fresh, ripe pawpaw (papaya)	All other fruit including dried fruit
Cereals	Rice, rice flour, rice noodles, rice biscuits, rice flakes, arrowroot, cornflour (wheat free)	All other cereals, bread, cakes, biscuits and related products
Sugars	White sugar (sucrose), rice syrup, golden syrup (all sugars should be used very sparingly)	Honey, maple syrup, molasses, artificial sweeteners, fructose, lactose
Condiments	Salt, fresh parsley	Herbs, spices, vinegar
Beverages	Water (purified if necessary), mineral water, pear nectar	Tea, coffee, alcoholic beverages, fruit drinks

Figure 3.9 (Cont'd)

Foods permitted		Foods disallowed
Medications and Toiletries	Consult with doctor Use salt (instead of toothpaste) and non-allergenic cosmetics	Aspirin, Disprin, Alka Seltzer or any drug containing aspirin, flavouring or colouring agents, cough syrups and lozenges, lotions, creams or rubs containing oil of wintergreen, methyl salicylate; other perfumes and cosmetics; vitamin supplements containing para amino benzoic acid (PABA), kelp, rosehips, alfalfa, yeast, colouring agents, lactose and other reactive excipients

Figure 3.10   **Sample menu for low chemical-reactant diet (Grade 1) (to be followed for a limited period of time until adverse reactions disappear; this usually takes 2–6 weeks)**

Breakfast	Lamb chops or Boiled egg Slice of pawpaw Rice Bubbles with pear nectar and sugar Water or pear nectar
Lunch	Chicken leg or breast Lettuce/parsley Rice biscuit Fresh pear (peeled) Mineral water
Dinner	Baked veal and potatoes (peeled) using sunflower oil
or	Grilled steak with boiled potatoes (peeled) Fresh lettuce Baked, peeled pear with cashew cream (blend raw cashews with a little water)
or	Pears in syrup Water or pear nectar

Note: This is an example of a strict elimination diet where one or more major food groups (e.g. dairy products) have been totally eliminated or severely restricted (e.g. fruit and vegetables). It is essential that appropriate low reactant nutrition supplements be taken whilst following this diet, especially a calcium tablet and perhaps a fibre supplement: hence, the importance of obtaining professional advice introduce new foods, in small amounts and one at a time. Each newly introduced food should be treated as a 'food challenge' and watched for possible adverse reactions. Both diets are intended to be a guide only, and should be discussed with either a medical practitioner, dietitian, nutritionist or natural health practitioner *who is familiar with the area of food and chemical sensitivities.* Many doctors and nutritionists working in this field introduce the suspected reactant chemicals as unmarked challenge capsules under double-blind conditions to rule out subjectivity when looking for positive reactions.

Figure 3.11 Low chemical-reactant diet (Grade 2: moderate)

Foods permitted		Foods disallowed
Meat and Eggs	Beef, veal, turkey, chicken, quail, venison, homemade hamburger mince, fresh pork fillet (trim off the fat), lamb sausages made with rice flour (selected butchers will make these without preservatives), brains, rabbit; fresh fish (not more than two days old), eggs; homemade soups and stocks	Bacon, ham, corned beef, frankfurters, meat pies, commercial sausages, canned meat and pastes, luncheon meats, sausage rolls, battered canned or bottled fish or other seafood; herrings, rollmops, canned oysters, etc.; commercially prepared egg products, custards, etc.
Dairy products and oils	*Minimum* quantities of cow's milk, natural yoghurt, buttermilk and ricotta cheese; plain additive-free butter and cream, copha, cold pressed safflower and sunflower oils	Ice cream, flavoured milks, artificial or longlife cream or milk, flavoured and fruit yoghurts, hard cheese and fermented cheeses (Camembert, blue vein, etc.), cheese spreads; all other oils with additives, commercial salad dressing
Vegetables	Artichokes, asparagus, (small portion), green beans, sprouts, brussels sprouts, cabbage, carrots (small portion) celery, chives, choko, cauliflower (small portion), corn, garlic, lettuce, leeks, legumes (dried — lentils, chick peas, dried beans in general) onions, sweet potato, swedes,	Chicory, capsicum, cucumber, chilli, endive, mushrooms, olives, gherkins, tomato, zucchini, peppers, okra, watercress, tinned baked beans, dried vegetables, eggplant, squash, broccoli, beetroot, radish, broad beans

Figure 3.11 (Cont'd)

Foods permitted		Foods disallowed
Vegetables (cont'd)	pumpkin, peas, parsley, turnip, marrow (small portion), spinach (small portion), shallots	
Fruit	Pears (without skin), pawpaws (papaya), mangoes, lemon (small quantities), lychees (small quantity) kiwi fruit (small quantity), custard apple, watermelon (small quantity), rockmelon, canteloupes (small piece)	Apples, apricots, avocado, bananas, blackberries, blackcurrants, blueberries, boysenberries, cherries, currants, cranberries, gooseberries, grapes, grapefruit, nectarines, oranges, peaches, plums, prunes, passionfruit, raisins, raspberries, rhubarb, redcurrants, strawberries, pineapple, dried fruit
Bread Cereals Grains	100 per cent rye bread; barley, oats, rice, millet, buckwheat, sago, tapioca, arrowroot, cornflour, potato flour, soya flour, Rice Bubbles, puffed rice, Corn Flakes, Popped rice (most cereals containing the above ingredients but without additives)	Breads or cereals containing fruits or colouring agents. Commercial cereals with a high sugar content, tinned spaghetti, wheat bread
Biscuits	Homemade using permitted ingredients	Commercial cakes and biscuits, cake mixes, puddings, instant desserts, pastries, dessert toppings, custard mixes
Beverages and Alcohol	Carob, Milo, Aktavite, Ovaltine (all made with 50% milk), pear nectar, camomile tea, mineral water, distilled spirits, whisky, gin, bacardi, vodka (½ nips)	Beer, wine, cider, liqueurs, port, cocoa, chocolate, milk shakes, all commercial soft drinks, cordials, and other fruit juices, coffee, tea
Nuts and Seeds	Cashews (raw, dry roasted) hazelnuts, macadamia, pecan, walnuts and brazil nuts in small amounts, sesame seeds, sunflower seeds, pumpkin seeds	Commercial snack nuts, almonds, peanuts, water chestnuts, pine nuts, pistachio nuts

Figure 3.11 (Cont'd)

Foods permitted		Foods disallowed
Condiments	Garlic, parsley (fresh), salt, soya sauce (Tamari), lemon juice, tahini (ground hulled sesame seeds)	Vegemite, Marmite, Bonox, Promite, other forms of soy sauce, vinegar (malt, wine and apple cider), fish paste, herbs, desiccated coconut, spices, fresh and dried mint, pickles, chutney, mustard, tomato sauce, other commercial sauces
Sugars	Carob, maple syrup, golden syrup, rice syrup, white sugar (sucrose), in small quantities	Artificial sweeteners, honey, flavoured syrups, jams, jellies
Medications	Plain unflavoured, uncoloured (white), toothpaste salt, clear capsules, white tablets, Panadol, Panadeine, Codeine	Aspirin, Disprin, Vincents, methyl salicylate (oil of wintergreen), coloured, flavoured vitamins and drugs. Check excipients (see Figure 3.5 on aspirin containing medication)

Figure 3.12   **Sample menu for low chemical-reactant diet (Grade 2)**

BREAKFASTS

1. Brown rice with maple syrup, soy milk and chopped hazelnuts. Pear juice.

2. Super drink (add egg, pear slices, maple syrup, spoonful of ground sesame or sunflower seeds to soy or cashew milk, and blend).
   Rice Bubbles or cornflakes with canned pears.

3. Sliced fresh pawpaw or pear juice.
   Homemade muesli (oats, rice bran, chopped hazelnuts, brazilnuts, toasted sesame and sunflower seeds). Golden syrup, yoghurt.

4. Pawpaw slices with lemon juice or fresh/canned mango slices.
   Eggs.
   100 per cent rye bread toast with butter (or hazelnut butter) and golden syrup.

5. Mango juice.
   Oats porridge with goats' yoghurt and golden syrup.

6. Rockmelon slices.
   Waffles or pancakes made from allowable flours (e.g. rice, cornmeal) with maple or golden syrup, hazelnut or cashew butter

Figure 3.12   (Cont'd)

7. Pawpaw slices (papaya).
   Bubble and squeak (reheated fried vegetables).
8. Mango slices.
   Corn on the cob.

DINNERS

1. Artichokes vinaigrette (cold pressed oil, lemon juice, garlic, parsley)

   Beef casserole (beef, onion, carrots, celery, garlic, parsley)
   Baked sweet potato
   Green beans or salad

   Baked pears with sago. Soy custard sweetened with arrowroot.

2. Fresh asparagus (tossed in butter and lemon juice)

   Roast veal
   Cauliflower in white sauce (thickened with arrowroot)
   Baked onion or chokos
   Green salad

   Watermelon balls

3. Celery soup (chicken stock, celery and turnip)

   Cabbage rolls (with mince and brown rice)
   Mashed pumpkin
   Green salad

   Jelly or flummery made with pear juice or mango juice and agar

4. Fresh oysters with 100 per cent rye bread and sprout salad (sprouts, grated carrot, shallots, parsley)

   Pork fillet stir-fried with cabbage, shallots, onions, carrot sticks, celery sticks, mung bean sprouts
   Brown rice

   Mango or custard apple

5. Braised leeks

   Vegetarian or salmon patties
   Spinach purée with lemon juice
   Corn cut off cob

   Stewed pear with cashew cream

6. Pumpkin soup

   Lamb chops or sausages
   Brown rice and carrot patties
   Cabbage salad (with celery, chives, walnuts, lemon vinaigrette)
   Rockmelon balls

Figure 3.12   (Cont'd)

7. Red lentil soup (cook with carrots, celery, onion, and purée)
   Roast turkey
   Baked pumpkin
   Peas
   Brussels sprouts
   Lychees or kiwi fruit

PACKED LUNCHES

1. Rice crackers with chick pea dip (hummus)
   Celery sticks
   Pears

2. Rye bread with salmon and lettuce
   Sliced rockmelon

3. Bean salad
   Hard-boiled egg
   Sliced pawpaw

4. Mango and chicken salad
   Nut and seed balls (ground nuts and seeds bound with a little nut butter
   and golden syrup)
   Pear

5. Rye bread with ricotta cheese, mixed with grated carrot, chopped celery
   Brazil nuts.

6. Corn on the cob
   Cold hamburger patties
   Kiwi fruit

7. Rice salad
   Cold sausages (rice flour, preservative free)
   Pear

8. Salmon patties
   Sliced pawpaw

Drink mineral water or camomile tea

4

Contaminants in our food supply

Antibiotic residues

For many years now farmers and other food producers have come to rely heavily on antibiotics to increase the growth rate of their food animals, thereby leading to a reduction in costs and also in the possible spread of disease in, for example, battery chickens. The concept of producing bigger, fatter animals much faster and cheaper, and with less disease, is very attractive to food producers. However, the use of subtherapeutic amounts of antibiotics in animal feed is not without its problems.

Bacteria and other microorganisms in animals have a remarkable ability to develop resistance to antibiotics and pass on this resistance genetically. It is transferred from organism to organism within and across species lines by packages of gene designated R factors residing on plasmids, the small circular pieces of DNA similar to those investigators use in recombinant DNA experiments. These units of DNA exist apart from the cell's chromosomes where most of the genetic material is located. Through a mating process the R factors pass from bacterium to bacterium, transferring the genetic information in a classic natural case of recombinant DNA. Although there is no direct evidence that these antibiotic-resistant bacteria are transmitted to people who eat meat or eggs from these animals, there is evidence that the genetic material contained in these plasmids may

certainly be transferred from animals that are eaten to humans.
There is also evidence that people who handle raw meat, or feed
laced with antibiotics, have a large number of resistant bacteria
in their gut. In 1976 the chief of the American Food and Drug
Administration, Donald Kennedy, said that although we can
point to no specific instance in which human disease is more
difficult to treat, because the drug resistance has arisen from an
animal source, it is likely that the problem could have gone
unnoticed. It has recently become front page news in South
Dakota and other places in the United States where people have
eaten hamburger mince derived from cattle that were fed subtherapeutic amounts of the antibiotic, chlortetracycline. These
very small amounts led to the production of *Salmonella newport*
resistant strains in the beef, and these or their plasmids were
then transferred through the hamburger beef to many people.
When some of these same people subsequently took a course of
antibiotics, all the pathogens in the gut were wiped out, with
the exception of the resistant *Salmonella newport*; as a result,
these resistant strains of *Salmonella* ran riot without the other
more friendly forms of gut microorganisms to hold them in
check. Many of these people ended up in hospital. So there is
now definite evidence that the use of small amounts of
antibiotics in animal feed for growth promotion and disease
prevention can indirectly affect the health of consumers. In the
past it was thought that the benefit of using these drugs in
animal feed far outweighed potential risks, but we may now
have to reconsider the situation.

    Added to these findings is almost universal agreement that
doctors are in general overprescribing antibiotics. As a result
there have developed many new strains of antibiotic resistant
bacteria such as methicillen resistant *Staphylococcus aureus*. Recently in Australian hospitals there have been a number of
serious outbreaks, leading to deaths, simply because the *Staphylococcus* was resistant to most forms of antibiotics. There is
much pressure all over the world on the medical profession at
the moment to reduce the prescription rate of antibiotics.
Special re-education programs have been directed at medical
practitioners to put an end to the random prescribing of
antibiotics for such passing maladies as the common cold but
the results of these remain to be seen.

The use of antibiotics for growth promotion and disease prevention in animals is only one aspect of a minor revolution that has gone on in the production of food animals in recent years, particularly in the United States. It has been suggested that the growth-promoting properties of antibiotics is seen only when animals are raised under suboptimal conditions in dirty, heavily contaminated pens, for instance, which are also over-crowded. Jim Mason from Missouri, and Peter Singer, Professor of Philosophy at Monash University in Melbourne, have recently published a book called *Animal Factories*, which puts into perspective the effects of the serious changes that are now occurring in the mass production of food animals. They write that animals are being placed in huge confined buildings instead of being free to run in pastures, that artificial lights and temperature controls are replacing sunlight and seasons and that concrete and metal confinement is all the animal can expect from birth to early death in the abattoirs. Economic expediency has largely replaced the need for healthy animals: as long as animals are big and fat and command a good price at market, all is assumed to be well. Whether the animal is high in protein or micronutrients does not seem to matter much any more. One would think that one of the top priorities in the production of food animals would be to have high-quality food for the animal, but even this is apparently not so. Cases are reported where pig farmers have allowed their cows to eat droppings froms hens housed above. One American farmer says that he doesn't have to feed his pigs for ninety days, thereby saving $9,300 each year on feed. To economise another farmer feeds his cattle on a diet of 75 per cent sawdust mixed with ammonia. In some factory farms raw poultry and pig manure is mixed with corn and stalks for pig and cattle feed, and animal waste is processed and sold as food supplements by agribusiness companies. Animal scientists are working on ways of channelling liquid wastes from factory manure kits and human wastes, back to animals. All these procedures are going to lead to the recycling of antibiotics and other additives in the already inadequate food supply of the animal.

Presently half of the antibiotics produced in the United States are used in animal feed. All farmers use them for poultry, 90 per cent for pigs, and veal calves, and 60 per cent for cattle. Singer

Table 4.1 Antibiotic resistant bacteria in Australian food animals

State of origin	Store/packager	Growth of bacteria isolated	Bacteria found	Antibiotics bacteria* resistant to	Probable source of contamination
			BEEF — TOPSIDE ROAST		
NSW	Woolworths	XXXX	staphylococci/ streptococci	penicillins/nr	handling
NT	Darwin Cheap Foods	XXXX	gm – ve rod	streptomycin, tetracyclines	handling
QLD	Woolworths	X	staphylococci	penicillins, tetracyclines	handling
SA	Farmland	X	staphylococci	penicillins	handling
TAS	Farmland	ng	ng	na	na
VIC	Farmland	X	staphylococci	penicillins, lincomycin	handling
WA	Farmer Direct	XXX	gm – ve rod	nitrofurantoin	handling
			PORK — PORK LEG		
NSW	Woolworths	X	gm – ve rod	nitrofurantoin	handling
NT	Darwin Cheap Foods	XXX	gm – ve rod	nitrofurantoin	handling
QLD	Woolworths	X	gm – ve rod	tetracyclines, streptomycin	handling
SA	Arkaba Village Meats	XXX	gm – ve rod	tetracyclines, streptomycin, nitrofurantoin	handling
TAS	Farmland	X	gm – ve rod	nr	handling
VIC	Farmland	XX	gm – ve rod	nitrofurantoin	handling
WA	Farmland	X	gm – ve rod	tetracyclines	handling

CHICKEN — COMMERCIAL

State	Company	Count	Organism	Antibiotic resistance	Source
NSW	Inghams Enterprises	XX	gm – ve rod	nitrofurantoin	intestinal tract
NT	Inghams Country Farm	XX	gm – ve rod	tetracyclines	intestinal tract
QLD	Golden Cockerel	XX	Proteus spp	tetracyclines, streptomycin, nitrofurantoin	intestinal tract
SA	Pape Bros Poultry Service	XXX	staphylococci/gm – ve rod	penicillins, chloramphenicol, lincomycin/tetracyclines	handling/intestinal tract
TAS	Golden Poultry Farming	XXXX	gm – ve	tetracyclines	intestinal tract
VIC	Mario's Poultry	XXX	E. coli	tetracyclines, streptomycin, nitrofurantoin	intestinal tract
WA	Table Talk Poultry	X	gm – ve rod	nitrofurantoin	intestinal tract

CHICKEN — DOMESTIC

State	Company	Count	Organism	Antibiotic resistance	Source
na	na	XX	staphylococci	nr	handling
na	na	X	gm + ve coccus	penicillins	handling

TURKEY — SELF BASTING

State	Company	Count	Organism	Antibiotic resistance	Source
NSW	Steggles	ng	ng	na	na
NSW	AA Tegel	X	gm – ve rod	tetracyclines, nitrofurantoin	intestinal tract

Source: Findings of the Australian Consumers Association published in *Choice* Magazine (December 1985)

na   not applicable (domestic chicken tested for comparative purposes only)
ng   no growth
nr   no resistance
gm – ve gram negative
gm + ve gram positive
spp   species
*   applies only to the antibiotics we tested for; other antibiotic resistance may also have been present

X   less than 20 colonies (insignificant)
XX   20 to 50 colonies
XXX   50 to 200 colonies
XXXX   more than 200 colonies (gross contamination)

and Mason have pointed out that in the past, contact with soil gradually exposed animals to a vast range of different bacteria and microorganisms allowing their natural immunity to work effectively. As they grazed in various parts of fields they would eat different varieties of the food they needed. They would also put their waste products back into the soil to enrich it without pollution. A good many animal producers have recently realised that by using caging houses and confining animals there is a general depression in food quality. As a result there has grown up a widespread use of 'compensatory' chemistry, to impart flavour, colour and other characteristics lost or depleted in the processing of the animals for food. When we consider how important it is for the average human to get daily exercise and our susceptibility to disease when we don't, or when we are under excessive stress, it requires little imagination to see how the quality of life for some of these food animals is going to directly and adversely affect the health of the animal.

For example, eggs that are derived from caged battery chickens may be lower in some nutrients such as B12 ánd folic acid, compared with eggs from free-ranging chickens. Over the years there has also been a slow increase in fat and water content in many of our animals such as chickens at the expense of good-quality protein. This is the direct result of the rapid growth-promoting techniques presently used. Singer and Mason further quote a veterinarian who became a meat inspector after twenty years of animal farm practice. He says: 'There are a number of major human diseases, namely cancer, heart disease and gallstones that ... originate in the meat packing plants of this country.' He claims that many of the animals that contract cancer are processed into pig and chicken feed and recycled back into the animal food chain. These new techniques of food production necessitate the use of antibiotics, steroids and colouring agents which come through the food line to adversely affect human behaviour and health. When a person complains of food intolerance, is that person really reacting to the food itself or is he or she fighting the remnants of sprays, drenches, hormones, antibiotics and other additives which have permeated the tissues of an animal during its preparation for the dinner table?

In spite of this dreary picture of Singer and Mason's, many of these problems have been recognised and acted upon in

Australia. The use of hormones in chicken production, for example, was banned in 1958, and antibiotics are now supposed to be used only when there is an outbreak of disease, and even then under strict veterinary supervision. Such controls are not always adhered to, but the Australian Chicken Meat Federation claims to produce birds which have natural resistance to many of the major poultry diseases by a process of cross-breeding different kinds of chickens. Due to genetic programming and carefully planned nutrition, Australian chickens are ready for eating after forty-two or forty-three days of life. They are fed pellets containing mostly wheatmeal, barley, sorghum, soya bean meal, meat meal for protein, as well as vitamins and minerals.

However, despite this reassurance *Choice* magazine (December 1985) spoke with Dr. Alan Frost, a senior pathologist at the University of Queensland who claimed that almost 100 per cent of commercially raised poultry in Australia is fed antibiotics at some stage of their growth, with 85 per cent of chickens carrying antibiotic resistant bacteria. Later, private laboratory tests carried out by *Choice* verified this claim. Every chicken examined contained intestinal bacteria resistant to at least one antibiotic used in human medicine (see Table 4.1). At the completion of testing, *Choice* said:

> We also tested all the meats for antibiotic residues — with some disturbing results. Five of 14 beef and pork samples contained residues of tetracyclines — used in human medicine — as did one of the two turkey samples. Residues in flesh show that the animals were treated with or fed antibiotics. All tetracycline residues were well above maximum levels allowed by the states and recommended by the World Health Organization.

5

Contamination of foods
with toxic minerals

Another area of concern is the possible contamination of our food supply with heavy metals and other toxic minerals. Those posing the greatest threat to human health are presently the minerals mercury, aluminium and lead. Let us take mercury as an example. When I was a boy it was that interesting heavy silver fluid which exploded into tiny droplets if you let it drop on a flat surface and merged into one big droplet if you gave it a little gentle coaxing. It was even more interesting if you considered the childhood stories of mad hatters in Paris who absorbed toxic mercury from hat bands, or the English noblewomen who used to take it orally to give them a fair (and deadly) complexion. Nowadays, the closest most people come to mercury in any great quantities is in the dentist's chair, where little blobs of mercury-based amalgam are neatly rammed into drilled out molars. Or, if you have a healthy set of ivories, you may have discovered that a daily thermometer is the best way of heralding the time of ovulation.

A more insidious aspect of mercury has emerged over recent years. The most prevalent biologically active form is called methyl mercury and it has now contaminated our food chain, particularly in fish and shellfish. Mercury also now enters our environment as the waste product of several industrial activities, and through organomercurial fungicides and from geographical sources, especially as a result of acid rain. Burning fossil fuels are also to blame, as are the refining of ores. It is also used as an integral part of paint, pulp, paper, cosmetics, pharmaceutical products and electrical equipment, all of them leading to the contamination of our drinking water and food supply.

The first indication that methyl mercury may become a potential problem in our foods arose in the 1950s and 1960s in Japan, where severe neurological damage was reported in several hundred individuals who had consumed fish contaminated with it. It had originated from industrial effluent released into Minamata Bay and also from Niigata. Further poisonings occurred in Iraq in 1960 and 1972 after wheat seed treated with methyl mercury antifungal agents had been ground into flour and used to make bread. Seven thousand people were affected and the mortality rate was around eight hundred. Symptoms of methyl mercury toxicity start with numbness and parasthesia around the mouth, fingers and toes, slurred speech, loss of peripheral vision, diminished hearing, awkward gait and incoordination. Animal experiments have revealed that 90 per cent of an orally administered dose of methyl mercury quickly finds its way into the body, where it binds to plasma proteins and to haemoglobin in red blood cells. It then attacks the blood-brain barrier, resulting in increased permeability of the brain, on one hand, and considerable dysfunction on the other, resulting in a reduced uptake of amino acids and metabolites by the central nervous system. The activities of many of the neurotransmitter enzymes are also reduced by it, i.e. the enzymes responsible for the production of the chemicals which relay nerve impulses from one part of the brain to another or from one nerve to a muscle are inactivated. In addition, the peripheral nervous system which supplies most of the muscles throughout our body and also relays sensory information back to the brain is a prime target. Many of these nerves, called axons, start to degenerate and both the nerve roots and trunks begin to lose their protective outer covering, the myelin sheath. Nerve impulses are slowed down and there is weakening in the skeletal muscles.

Methyl mercury also affects the foetus and the neonate. Infants born to mothers who have been only mildly exposed and have shown no symptoms at all, still exhibit exaggerated muscle tone and tendon reflexes, ataxia, incoordination, involuntary movements, prolongation of primitive reflexes and delays in motor and psychological development. Tissue culture systems have shown that methyl mercury inhibits nerve migration in the developing human foetal cerebrum (the brain). There is a definite relationship between the frequency of neurological abnormalities in infants and the maximum maternal mercury hair levels during pregnancy. Mothers with maximum hair mercury levels in the range 99–384ppm were more likely to have infants with abnormal neurological findings compared with mothers whose hair mercury levels were less than 85ppm.

Based on evidence from Japan, the lowest estimated blood mercury concentration at which toxicity occurred was 0.2 micrograms per gram or 200 parts per billion. In order to calculate an appropriate 'action level' that would safeguard the consumer as well as the fishing industry the Food and Drug Administration arrived at a maximum daily mercury intake of 0.4 micrograms per kilogram body weight i.e. recommending that the average daily fish intake should not contain more than 1ppm of mercury. This, of course, assumes that there are no other major dietary sources of mercury and that the body's mechanism for removing it are adequate. Unfortunately, the renal and biliary systems, the main excretory systems for methyl mercury, are not fully developed in the neonate, hence the newborn infant may not be able to remove it as efficiently as an adult. This may be a highly relevant point, as methyl mercury contamination in the mother is easily transferred through the placenta to the foetus, and is also delivered via the breast milk. Its concentration in breast milk has been found to be the same as maternal blood levels.

While daily exposure to mercury for most of us is nowhere near as great as that found in Japan during the 1960s, there is always the problem of a slow accumulation of mercury in the liver and brain cells. Even though it has a biological half-life of seventy-four days, it is still known that the removal of heavy metals from the nervous system occurs much more slowly than for other tissues. Also, although the overall distribution of mercury in the foetus is similar to that found in the adult, it appears that foetal brain levels are relatively higher than those found in the adult. In view of the inefficient mechanisms in the foetus and the neonate for removal of mercury, even small background exposure levels transferred to the foetus may have lasting effects on the blood-brain-barrier, the metabolic processes and cellular membranes of the infant's nervous system leading, perhaps, to sensory, motor and behaviour disturbances.

In later life amalgam fillings may present another toxic source of mercury for many individuals. While such mercury is not exactly present in the food, the act of chewing food greatly increases its release from the filling. Amalgam is an unstable alloy and continously gives off mercury in the form of gas, ions and abraded particles. The level of mercury present in respired air from fillings one week and two years old alike is about 2.8 micrograms/m^3 (14ng/10 breaths). After irritation by, say, chewing gum this level increases sharply to about 40 micrograms/m^3. People are especially at risk of exposure when fillings are removed, and there should be a powerful air suction to protect both the patient and the dentist during such dental work. The patient should avoid swallowing amalgam powder or pieces and dental work should be delayed if open wounds are present in the oral cavity.

One researcher examining the slow loss of mercury from amalgam fillings showed that the amount of mercury missing from an outer corroded zone (50–90 micrometers) was equivalent to about 560mg in a mouth containing many fillings. This represents a loss of 150 micrograms a day over a ten year period. In addition, amalgam fillings with time become porous, increasing the surface area greatly and enhancing corrosion. Corrosion in some extracted teeth is reportedly so severe that most of their strength has been lost and they can easily be crushed with the fingers. Corrosion of amalgam is also the main cause for failure of fillings.

American gynaecologists say that fertile women should not be exposed to mercury vapour levels higher than 10 micrograms/m^3 and pregnant women not to any raised levels at all, as the vapour passes quickly to the foetus and is excreted in milk during lactation.

In recent years another factor has started to contribute to the environmental pollution with heavy metals. This is the phenomenon called 'acid rain'. Fumes from car exhausts, and industrial gases that pour out of huge smoke-stacks contain sulphur and nitrogen oxides. These gases react with the water in the air to form sulphuric and nitric acids which fall to the ground as acid rain; this affects plant and animal life. It can affect human health in three ways: by deposition on the skin, through inhalation and by toxic effects from leaching various heavy metals from the earth's crust into our water and food supplies. At the moment there seems to be no great cause for alarm about acid rain settling on our skin. However, we have already raised the issue of sulphur dioxide inhalation for chronic asthmatic patients. Many such patients living in polluted areas react to the sulphur dioxide in the air with upper respiratory distress, wheezing and frequently, asthma attacks: acid rain can produce acute and chronic respiratory damage. In addition the sulphate or sulphuric acid that is also formed in the polluted air tends to hamper the clearance of toxins which accumulate daily in the lung. This effect appears to be related to the mucous lining of the bronchial tubes becoming acidified.

The most obvious effects of acid rain have been demonstrated by the disastrous impact it has had on some of the major forests of Europe and North America. Two thirds of the Black Forest in West Germany has been destroyed because of the effects of acid rain. Other flora and fauna have died in streams, rivers, and lakes. Its deadly effect seems to be due not only to its acidity, but also to its ability to mobilise minerals from the ground including cadmium, manganese, nickel, zinc and, more relevant to our discussion, mercury, aluminium, and lead. An increased concentration of these three toxic minerals has been found in the water running off geographically sensitive areas.

We are already most concerned about the problem of city children having higher blood lead levels affecting learning ability and performance at school. Children absorb more lead than adults, and retain a much higher percentage in their bodies. The usual intake comes from three sources: air, dust and food. Probably the major source is the exhaust gases of cars burning leaded petrol. If the fumes are not directly inhaled the lead settles in the dust, and this, particularly on the sides of roads, is one of the great sources of lead ingestion for children, who of course play close to the ground. The enamel coating of cheap plates and other eating utensils imported from the Third World can be another minor contributing source of lead. Recently we have come to understand that drinking water may be another major source of lead ingestion, and can be a significant contributor to increased blood lead levels. Acid rain not only increases human exposure to lead by leaching it from soils and rocks, but also has the effect of lowering the pH of domestic water supplies, making drinking water more acidic. Where city water supplies have a high acidic content, usually with a pH less than 6.5, as occurs at the moment in Glasgow, Scotland, which has a domestic water pH in the vicinity of 6.3, blood lead levels are high in the population drinking that water. When the same water is treated in some way or alkalised so that the pH rises to pH9 there is a significant reduction in blood lead levels.

There is now general agreement that atmospheric lead fallout is the major source of lead in typical food crops consumed by humans and farm animals, and this originates from petrol. A study of the lead levels on both inner and outer leaves of cabbages in the Reading area of Britain revealed up to 8ppm in outer leaves 50 feet from the roadside and 5ppm in leaves grown 650 feet from the road. Airborne lead contributed 90 per cent of the total in exposed leaves. In Denmark, atmospheric lead settling on the surface of leaves of grass constitutes between 90 and 99 per cent of the total lead content of the pastures: food and airborne lead are no longer independent variables. This finding applies not only to vegetable and cereal crops consumed by humans, but also to meat. Consumption of grass contaminated by aerial fallout of lead, together with inhalation of lead by sheep and cattle, gives rise to most of the lead surfacing in the animals' flesh and organs.

A recent study in Zurich examined the lead in 172 different vegetable samples grown in the town. It was concluded that the lead values were significantly higher than in country-grown vegetables. In New Zealand the lead concentrations in vegetation and soil next to a road carrying over 23,000 vehicles a day decreased exponentially with distance from the road, from 197 and 262 micrograms of lead per gram at 4.2 metres, to 8 and 23 micrograms per gram for vegetation and soil, respectively, at 300 metres from the roadside. The investigator making these measurements also felt that continuous grazing of sheep close to the road could result in high concentrations of lead in liver and kidney tissues, so that people eating kidney and liver would gain high levels of lead. It is now well known that bone meal supplements sold in health food stores frequently have high levels of lead for this reason.

Current estimates of lead/calcium ratios in the bones of

Table 5.1   Comparison of estimated natural levels of lead in the environment with typical present-day levels

Medium	Estimated natural lead concentration	Typical present-day lead concentrations	Approximate ratio present day/natural
Air			
rural/remote	0.01–0.1 ng/m^3	0.1–100 ng/m^3	10–1,000
inhabited	0.1–1.0 ng/m^3	0.1–10 μg/m^3	100–10,000
Soil			
rural/remote	5–25 μg/g	5–50 μg/g	1–2
inhabited	5–25 μg/g	10–5,000 μg/g	2–200
Water			
fresh	0.005–10 μg/1	0.005–10 μg/1	1
ocean	0.001 μg/1	0.005–0.015 μg/1	10
Foods	0.0001–0.1 μg/g	0.01–10 μg/g	100

Source: From United States National Academy of Sciences Report

residents living in Britain and the United States are about 100–500 times greater than in bones uncovered in Peru buried about 1,600 years ago. The United States National Academy of Sciences has estimated that we now have a 100 times increase in typical lead concentrations in foods compared with what used to exist in natural foods before industrial contamination (see Table 5.1).

Unfortunately once lead pollutes the soil there is no way of removing it. It doesn't break down into a less toxic mineral, and it does not decay. The lead in soil and human bones just accumulates.

Probably the world's expert in lead and health, Dr. D. Bryce-Smith, has observed that: the FAO/WHO maximum intake for adults is equivalent to 430 micrograms of lead per day in the diet. For the 'standard' 70kg man, this is equivalent to about 6 micrograms/kg/day in round figures. The WHO maximum is specifically based on an assumed 10 per cent gastrointestinal absorption rate, so since the rate for children is now known to be some five times higher, a corresponding maximum for them would be one fifth of the adult rate, i.e. 1.2 micrograms/kg/day, say 1 microgram/kg/day in round figures, to make some allowance for the greater sensitivity of the less mature organism. By comparison dietary intakes measured for bottle fed infants ranged up to thirty times this, with an average of 3 micrograms/kg/day. 'Normal' children, aged 3 months to 8½ years and 2 weeks to 2 years, showed average absorption rates of 53 and 43 per cent respectively, and corresponding dose rates of 10.61 and 10.29 micrograms/kg/day, some ten times greater than the FAO/WHO equivalent maximum deduced above, and nearly double the maximum for adults.

These calculations indicate that the majority of young children in Britain today, and certainly in other industrialised societies, are already exposed to grossly elevated intakes of dietary lead. How quickly the change to lead-free petrol will tend to reverse this situation remains to be seen. Such action is not before time in view of the numerous studies associating subtoxic lead levels in children with hyperactivity, impulsiveness, short attention span, negative ratings by teachers on classroom behaviour, school failure due to behavioural and learning problems, mental disorders and recently, emotional disturbances. In the case of 37 emotionally disturbed children and 107 normal control children, the disturbed group exhibited significantly higher levels of hair lead (5.67ppm [p < 0.001] versus controls 2.76ppm) and mercury (0.96ppm [p < 0.01] versus controls 0.47ppm). Discriminant function analysis revealed that by using lead, mercury as well as arsenic and aluminium levels, subjects could be correctly classified as disturbed with 77.8 per cent accuracy. Analyses also revealed significant positive correlations between lead and the Walker Problem Behaviour Identification Checklist (WPBIC) scales, measuring acting out, withdrawal, distractibility, disturbed peer relations and immaturity: there were significant positive correlations between mercury and acting out, disturbed peer relations and immaturity. The investigators performing this study (Marlowe, et al) made the comment that even small quantities of the above heavy metals now appear to be associated with emotional disturbances in children.

A similar study by the same investigators has also shown that childhood mental retardation is related to the presence in the body of above normal levels of a whole range of minerals, especially lead and cadmium.

We have already spoken of the dangers of mercury fungicide treated seed grains and of eating fish exposed to industrial discharges such as happened in Japan. Acid rain could also promote an accumulation of methyl mercury in fish as a direct

Figure 5.1

Dangers of using primitively produced lead-glazed pottery from the Middle East

---

The cooking and storage of food in lead-glazed pottery produced by traditional methods from primitive kilns in Middle Eastern countries (especially Lebanon, Syria and Jordan) constitute a potential health hazard, warn a team of scientists headed by A. Acra from the Department of Environmental Health, Faculty of Health Sciences, American University of Beirut, Lebanon.

Tests performed on a variety of commercially produced lead glazed pottery utensils in Lebanon showed that lead is leached (over 24 hours by 4 per cent acetic acid) in significantly higher proportions from rural and primitively prepared types of pottery than from pottery prepared by modern controlled methods in Beirut and other countries. 'The mean value for the lead leached from the 275 utensils produced in the primitive potteries was 97.67mg/l (range 0.3 to 200mg/l), and only about 15 per cent complied with the maximum limit of 7.0mg/l of extracted lead set by the US Food and Drug Administration.'

Lemon juice and vinegar (in foods such as tabbouleh, fattoush, hommos, and fúl), yoghurt and pickles are traditionally widely consumed in these countries. Plumbism is therefore not inconceivable when the foods are prepared and stored in inadequately glazed utensils. As well, the researchers warn that workers in primitive potteries may be exposed to an occupational health hazard from lead, although extensive analysis of pottery workers has not been carried out. It is recommended that pottery prepared with a glaze of unfritted red lead (Pb_2O_4) be considered unfit for glazing domestic utensils, that the design and operation of existing and unsatisfactory rural kilns be modified, and that safer fritted lead glazes or lead-free glazes be used for food utensils. The researchers also feel that the soldered seams of cans containing such foods as hommos and fúl may leach lead into the food.

Lancet 1, 433–4 (1981)

---

consequence of acidifying surface waters. It can effectively remove mercury vapour from the atmosphere. The mercury can accumulate in fresh water, either from dry or wet precipitation, or indirectly from the run off of soils. Inorganic mercury undergoes changes when it is in the water sediment, bacteria tending to methylate the mercury, making a more toxic organic form, either by forming monomethyl or dimethyl mercury. The rate of the methylation process of mercury by microorganisms is dependent on how acid the water is: the more acid, the easier it is for mercury to be methylated.

Methyl mercury will accumulate in aquatic food chains with high muscle tissue concentrations in fish. The highest of these have been found in predatory fish such as lake trout, pike and bass. High tissue levels of methyl mercury (in fish muscle) have been correlated with the acidic pH of remote lake waters that are not contaminated by industrial sources. While there have not been any reported cases of poisoning from people eating methyl mercury-contaminated predatory fish in the area of lakes, it is certainly another source of food contamination.

Another potentially lethal metal that is leached out of the soil by acid rain is aluminium. In high acid rain fallout areas mobilisation of aluminium results in high concentrations in both surface and ground water. Again, the acid rain can be lethal to fish, not because of the acidification process but because of the increased content of aluminium. The toxicity of the aluminium depends on the particular species of fish as well as the concentration in it. Aluminium has also been implicated as an important factor in some neurological disorders, particularly in patients on chronic renal dialysis. Elderly psychiatric patients with the highest levels of aluminium in their hair have also been shown to be those with the greatest short term memory loss. Sohler et al found that the mean blood aluminium level for 120 individuals suffering from memory loss was 39.4ppb as compared to 272 individuals without memory loss whose mean was 31.3ppb. Many elderly patients take aluminium-containing antacids on a daily basis. One wonders whether this daily ingestion of huge quantities by the elderly population may in fact be contributing to presenile dementia and dementia itself.

The three areas of the world that presently have the highest aluminium level in their soils — Guam, the Ki Peninsula in Japan, and north west New Guinea — not only have a high aluminium level in their soils, but very low levels of calcium and magnesium. In these same areas there is a very high incidence of a motor neurone disorder called amyotrophic lateral sclerosis (ALS), and also Parkinsonism and Parkinson's Dementia, which may prove to be aluminium related. Chronic environmental deficiency of both calcium and magnesium also appears to favour increased intestinal absorption of aluminium

Figure 5.2

Environmental sources of aluminium
Aluminium pots, pans, cans and foil
Water supplies — aluminium flocculating agents employed in purification
Hot water supplies — cathodic corrosion prevention using aluminium cores
Baking powders
Spices
Food additives (sodium aluminium phosphate, emulsifier in cheese (aluminium calcium silicate); anticaking agent added to salt (potassium aluminium bleaching agent)
Pharmaceutical preparations:
Antacids (containing aluminium)
Bufferin
Aluminium hydroxide gels
Antiperspirants, deodorants
Airborne contamination from:
Air conditioner corrosion
Clay dust

and its subsequent deposition in the central nervous system.

Another disease that is at present rife among the elderly is Alzheimer's Disease. It affects about 5 per cent of the population who are aged more than sixty-five, and is one of the most common forms of mental deterioration in the elderly. Patients with Alzheimer's Disease have significant reductions in the activity of an enzyme in the brain called choline acetyl transferase. Aluminium has been shown to inhibit choline transport in erythrocytes (red blood cells) and also to decrease nerve tissue choline acetyl transferase activity. It is interesting that the brain tissue of patients with Alzheimer's Disease shows accumulation of aluminium, particularly in areas of the brain having a high percentage of neurons containing neurofibrillory tangles. It doesn't require much imagination to see that the acid rain problem that is occurring in Europe and North America that has already killed off much of the Black Forest and other vegetation in Europe, together with other environmental sources of aluminium, may be causing problems in the human nervous system by increasing the content of toxic minerals in daily food supplies and drinking water. So insidious is the problem that a

Figure 5.3

Aluminium preparations affect joint tissues
Aluminium has been found in high concentrations in the joint tissues of a 48-year-old man who had been on haemodialysis for chronic kidney failure and who had taken 4–10 grams aluminium hydroxide daily for five years. The patient required a total hip prosthesis because of the development of osteonecrosis of the left femoral head. During the operation samples of surrounding synovial tissue and cartilage exhibited aluminium levels 3 or 4 times greater than samples taken from patients that had not previously taken aluminium preparations. The synovial fluid sample showed 87 μg/l aluminium compared to control levels of 10.8 μg/l. These results indicate that aluminium ingestion may lead to a toxic reaction in joint tissues.
Letter, *Lancet* 8228, 1, 1056–7 (1981)

Figure 5.4

Aluminium toxicity in infants
Aluminium intoxication has been reported in three infants with azotaemia who were treated with aluminium hydroxide (>100mg elemental aluminium) since 4 weeks of age. Serum aluminium levels and daily dose of elemental aluminium were positively correlated and bone biopsies demonstrated osteomalacia and massive deposition of aluminium in bone. These findings reveal that aluminium hydroxide can be absorbed through the gastrointestinal tract leading to aluminium intoxication in children.
(Andreoli, S.P. *et al.* Aluminium intoxication from aluminium-containing phosphate binders in children with azotaemia not undergoing dialysis.) *N. Engl. J. Med.* 310 (17): 1079–84 (1984)

recent report in the *Lancet* demonstrates that even infant milk formulas are at risk.

In 1983, progressive encephalopathy (dysfunction and degeneration of the brain) was reported by researchers in twenty of twenty-three children with impaired kidney function who were *not* subjected to renal dialysis. Nor had they received any aluminium salts before symptoms developed. These observations pointed to another source of environmental aluminium contamination for children with chronic renal insufficiency: infant milk formulas. A recent report cites two infants with congenital uraemia (kidney disease) who had not received

118

Table 5.2   Aluminium content of milk formulas

Milk Formula	Aluminium (ng/ml)
Emfamil Premature Formula (24Kcal/oz)	391
Emfamil Neonatal (13Kcal/oz)	316
Similac Special Care (24Kcal/oz)	294
Similac Special Care (20Kcal/oz)	277
Similac PM 60/40 (20Kcal/oz)	232
Similac PM 60/40 powder mixed with Nursett water at full strength	208
Similac (24Kcal/oz)	208
Similac (20Kcal/oz)	126
Emfamil with Iron Formula (20Kcal/oz)	124
Breast milk	4
Nursett water	4

Note: These findings raise the possibility that the use of infant formulas may also pose an aluminium related health hazard for infants with normal kidney function
Source: Freundlich and co-workers (1985)

Table 5.3   Aluminium content (μg/l) of milk and intravenous fluids

Oral (locally reconstituted*)	Content	Intravenous	Content
Osterfeed (baby milk)	94	Water for injection BP	128
Osterfeed' (complete formula)	226	15% KCl (Phoenix)	225
SMA white cap	88	10% calcium gluconate	
SMA gold cap	92	(Phoenix)	3430
Cow and Gate (baby milk plus)	125	13.6% Potassium acid	
Cow and Gate (premium)	142	phosphate (McCarty)	1882
Wysoy	330	Dextrose 50% (Evans)	238
		Ped-el	1740
		Vitalipid	307
Oral (ready constituted)		Intralipid 10%	9
		Solvito	69
Nenatal	499	Standard Viaflex saline and	
Prematalac	168	dextrose solution	<1
Vamin 9 glucose	44		

* Constituted with local water (35 μg/l A1)
Source: McGraw, Bishop and O'Hara (1986)

aluminium-containing agents or intravenous fluids but who had died at one and three months respectively, after the sudden onset of neurological symptoms. Brain aluminium concentration was high in both infants and both were fed Similac PM 60/40. Analysis of the powdered milk formula revealed an aluminium level of 232ng/ml, with less than 4ng/ml present in the sterilised water used to make up the formula and also in the dialysate concentrate.

The aluminium content of other milk formulas was subsequently examined and also found to contain high levels of aluminium, as also were intravenous fluids (see Tables 5.2 and 5.3).

6

The question of fluoridation

In Western Europe there is widespread rejection of fluoridation and plants that have been in operation for many years are now closed. Countries that have rejected fluoridation include Austria, Belgium, Denmark, France, Greece, Holland, Italy, Luxemburg, Norway, Spain, Sweden, West Germany and Yugoslavia. Presently less than 8 per cent of Britain's population drinks fluoridated water. In the United States also, hundreds of cities have now rejected fluoridation.

In Australia, the proportion of the population drinking fluoridated water is now probably higher than in any other country. The Health (Fluoridation) Act decrees that the level to which fluorides are to be built up is to a maximum 'average optimum concentration' of 1ppm fluoride (Victorian Government 1973). Regulating the concentration at the taps of the consumers, however, is almost impossible, and most countries using fluoride report wide variations in such concentrations. In thirteen fluoridated American cities levels vary from 0 to 1.6ppm. fluoride. In Melbourne, Australia, fluoride concentrations have been reported at levels up to 2.6ppm. The sodium silicofluoride slurry used in Melbourne destroys steel pipes and causes marked corrugation of pipes. Similar encrustation of pipes in Seattle, Washington, in the United States, revealed 1,044ppm fluoride on inner surfaces which can break away to block filter systems.

Until recently many people living in Melbourne did not realise that their water was being fluoridated and many were still administering fluoride tablets to their children and using fluoridated toothpastes. As a result, many reports of fluorosis or

120

'mottled teeth' in children have surfaced. In 1977 the Council on Dental Therapeutics advised that children under two years of age should not take fluoride tablets containing more than 0.25mg per day (many were formerly taking 1.0mg tablets) due to the risk of fluorosis.

Sources of fluoride other than water supplies include food. Fluoride is present in nearly every food, with the highest concentrations found in tea, seafood, bone meal, spinach and gelatin. It is estimated that widespread use of fluoridated water (1ppm) in food processing and preparation will probably mean a food fluoride intake of approximately 1.0–1.2mg per day. In Britain a strong cup of tea was found to contain up to 0.3mg of fluoride. Fluoride is taken up by vegetables and plants when fluoridated town water supplies are used for irrigation and when superphosphate fertilisers and agricultural sprays containing fluoride are applied to fruits and vegetables. Some plants such as spinach (28.3ppm), and lettuce and parsley (both 11.3ppm) are fluorine accumulators. In one district in Japan the fluoride content of wheat rose by 64 per cent, of pumpkin by 429 per cent and in watermelons 831 per cent over a seven year period, mainly due to the use of fertilisers. In 1976 the United States Environmental Protection Agency set a tolerance limit of 7ppm of combined fluorine residues arising from insecticide fluorine compounds, cryolite and synthetic cryolite (sodium aluminium fluoride) for forty-nine different varieties of vegetables and fruits, as it was feared that higher amounts in fruit and vegetables would cause mild mottling of the enamel of children's teeth even with no fluorine in the drinking water.

When Valencia orange trees are exposed to hydrogen fluoride gas with a fluoride concentration of 1ppb there is a reduction in leaf size, total leaf surface area and a reduced top weight which is directly related to total fluoride accumulation. Some people are presently concerned about the effect of watering trees with water containing 1ppm fluoride, a thousand times the above concentration. Fluoridated water (1ppm) also reduces the keeping quality of cut flowers by about 20 per cent. There is also some concern that various species of plants are capable of making fluoroacetic acid (a fluorine containing organic acid) which is readily converted in the body into fluorocitric acid which poisons respiration in cells.

The actual toxicity of fluoride added to town water depends much upon the 'hardness' of the water, that is, the concentration of mainly calcium and magnesium. Calcium is the accepted antidote for fluoride poisoning, and lime water or calcium chloride solutions are used to wash out the stomach, or calcium gluconate injected intravenously. The higher the calcium and magnesium content of the water supply the lower will be the induced toxicity of the fluoride. It is possible to produce mottling and brown stains in the teeth of animals simply by lowering their dietary calcium intake below the need for growing animals. It is also possible to prevent mottling by supplying the normal calcium requirement of the animal. The lower the calcium status of the community in general, the more prevalent and severe is the mottling of teeth caused by fluoridation in the water supply. One undernourished Italian town with 1.3ppm fluoride in its water supply produced mottled teeth in 60 per cent of its inhabitants compared with a better nourished town in Illinois in the United States with the same fluoride content but producing an incidence of only 25.3 per cent mottled teeth. It may be highly significant that Melbourne's water supply is particularly soft with a calcium content of only 1.6ppm compared with many United States towns which usually range from 35–60ppm.

As naturally fluoridated waters are usually 'hard' and the fluoride ion concentrations in such systems are rarely greater than 0.1ppm, Melbourne is one city that may have an exceptional health risk associated with the fluoridation of its water supply at a level of 1ppm. With recent reports of an association between repetitive strain injuries (RSI) and the consumption of fluoridated water, it is interesting to consider the conclusions of a report submitted to the Committee of Inquiry into the Fluoridation of Victorian Water Supplies by Philip Sutton, Academic Associate at the University of Melbourne in 1980. His conclusions may be summarised as follows:

1. Fluoridation has been promoted by: (a) valueless 'endorsements' by various organisations, based mainly on hearsay (b) the repression of the opponents of fluoridation, and (c) the suppression of new evidence against it.
2. Fluoridation compulsorily medicates every member of the community through their domestic drinking water with

small doses of a poisonous substance. It contravenes medical ethics and may violate religious and personal convictions. It should not be confused with chlorination, which is intended to treat the water, not the consumer.

3. Claims that artificial fluoridation will reduce the number of dentists required by the community have not been proved.

4. There is an increasing rejection of fluoridation overseas. In Western Europe, plants which had been in operation for many years have been closed and there is now an almost complete rejection of fluoridation.

5. Opposition to fluoridation is expressed in most of the letters on the subject sent to the *Medical Journal of Australia*.

6. The concentration of fluoride in the domestic tap is very difficult to regulate and usually it is not at the specified level.

7. It has been necessary to add lime to the Melbourne water to combat the 'severe corrosion' which fluoride produces in water pipes.

8. Recent publications suggest that increasing the alkalinity of water, by adding lime, may be hazardous unless the water is also chlorinated.

9. Claims that fluoridation will produce a marked decrease (approximately 60 per cent) in the prevalence of dental caries have proved to be, at least, grossly exaggerated.

10. Dental fluorosis, due to chronic fluoride poisoning of tooth-forming cells, will occur in at least 10 per cent of children who drink fluoridated water from the time of birth.

11. The 'optimum' or 'optimal' fluoride concentration in drinking water (said to be approximately 1ppm) is the one which promoters of fluoridation consider is the most favourable one for teeth — they rarely consider its effect on the rest of the body.

12. Fluoride is being ingested in increasing quantities from sources other than water — from food, toothpaste and from fluoride pollution of the atmosphere. Little is known of the fluoride levels in the Melbourne air for the Environment Protection Authority does not monitor it.

13. There cannot be an 'optimum' total fluoride level for every member of a community for this value varies with each individual.

14. The important factor of temperature variations between

seasons has been ignored when fluoridating our water.

15. The fluoride concentration of drinking water which is specified in the Act is an arbitrary one.

16. Despite the addition of lime to Melbourne's waters they are still exceptionally 'soft', with low concentrations of calcium which is the antidote to fluoride poisoning.

17. Recent publications suggest the possibility that cases of skeletal fluorosis may develop in Victoria, particularly in those who live near fluoride-emitting factories.

18. Little is known of the psychological reactions of individuals afflicted with dental fluorosis, nor of the direct effects of fluoride on the central nervous system.

19. Recent discoveries give support to the finding that an increase in mongoloid births is associated with increasing levels of fluoride in water supplies.

20. Fluoridated water, apart from affecting the teeth, may have severe effects on other organs of the body. It should not be used in kidney dialysis machines.

21. It is now definitely established that some people cannot tolerate fluoridated drinking water. They become ill, but recover when distilled water is substituted for their domestic water for drinking and cooking.

22. Claims that there is a large margin of safety with fluoridation are false and 'patently naïve'.

23. Fluoridation introduces a 'fluoride circuit' which has an uncontrollable effect on man and his environment.

24. Despite claims to the contrary, the reported link between artificial fluoridation and increased cancer mortality has not been disproved. On the contrary, preliminary data from Birmingham, Britain, strongly support the presence of such a link.

7

Chemical exposure during pregnancy and breast feeding

Two very important areas to examine in any serious study of the impact of chemicals in foods on health, are pregnancy and breast feeding. The most important time for optimal nutrient intake for any individual is during pregnancy and lactatation, and excessive intakes of drugs and other foodborne chemicals can seriously interfere with rapid growth stages. During early pregnancy the embryonic cells differentiate into specific tissues and organs. The fertilised egg rapidly divides into many undifferentiated cells which become three main layers. Two inner layers, the endoderm and the mesoderm, become internal organs, bones, muscles and glands. The outer layer, the ectoderm, develops into nose, hair, nervous system, the lining of the gut, ducts for glands (such as breast, thyroid, pancreas) and also the skin.

One of the most important considerations during toxicological studies involving new drugs and food additives, and accidental or unavoidable environmental chemicals such as pesticides and herbicides, is the possibility that a newly introduced chemical may adversely effect the growth of the foetus, that is, it may be 'teratogenic'. There is also the other possibility, that it may affect future generations by interfering with the genetic material in the reproductive cells, in which case the

125

chemical becomes 'mutagenic'. There are many animal studies that demonstrate the teratogenic effects of inadequate nutrient status. When the growing embryo is deprived of essential amino acids (derived from protein) or essential fatty acids (derived from animal fat or vegetable oils) by feeding the mother diets deficient in the macronutrients, congenital abnormalities appear in the offspring. Even a modest reduction in the amount of essential oils or fats can adversely affect the formation of brain and nervous tissue in the foetus. This results in irreversible learning and behaviour problems in later life. Similar problems arise when the growing foetus is limited in a plentiful supply of micronutrients. These are the vitamins and minerals that are so critical for the formation and optimum function of new tissues and organs. Deficiency in any of the B vitamins, folic acid, riboflavin, niacin or thiamine or critical minerals such as magnesium, calcium, zinc, manganese and copper may result in congenital abnormalities including cleft palates, webbing of feet, holes in the heart, spina bifida or kidney or liver abnormalities. Scientific investigations have shown that women who have given birth to one or more children with a neural tube defect such as spina bifida have a significantly lower incidence of such abnormalities in subsequent children if they take a balanced low-dose multivitamin and mineral supplement throughout subsequent pregnancies. At-risk women who fail to take extra micronutrients demonstrate a significantly higher incidence of children with congenital abnormalities compared to those who take supplements. The first twelve weeks when new organs are forming in the foetus are especially critical and many congenital problems can often be traced back to acutely stressful periods: days without eating, planned fasting, extensive radiation therapy or drug therapy, environmental exposure to herbicides or other chemicals.

Many drugs have been shown to be teratogenic and the thalidomide tragedy has made gestational medication a very sensitive area. According to many animal studies the main reason for a drug's teratogenicity resides in its ability either to interact directly with essential micronutrients or to interfere with their absorption, distribution, storage and excretion. In this respect the deleterious effects of thalidomide in follow-up animal studies have been circumvented by increasing the experimental animals' status of zinc and certain relevant B vitamins.

Foetal Alcohol Syndrome, the congenital abnormality found in the offspring of women who have consumed excessive amounts of alcohol during their pregnancy, is also possibly related to an alcohol-induced depletion of essential micronutrients, especially folic acid, thiamine, riboflavin, pyridoxine, and the minerals, zinc and magnesium.

Studies of the coffee-drinking habits of Americans have revealed that both men and women now drink in excess of two cups per day. There has always been some concern that pregnant women may be at risk, because animal studies have revealed that caffeine can induce birth defects in high doses. Japanese researchers have found between 6 and 20 per cent of birth defects in litters after pregnant mice have been injected with 100–200mg/kg of caffeine. Other similar studies in Germany, France and England have also shown that birth defects occurred in 1–3 per cent of the offspring in two studies, but none in a third when caffeine was fed orally to pregnant mice in amounts corresponding to twenty-five cups of coffee a day. Malformations in animals have included limb reduction deformities, cleft palates, and subcutaneous haemorrhages, but to equate these results with the human situation, a pregnant woman would have to drink over twenty-five cups of coffee each day during pregnancy, which is highly unlikely. During a more realistic study of the coffee-drinking habits of 800 Utah and Idaho women, most of whom were non-coffee and non-alcohol drinking members of the Church of Jesus Christ of Latterday Saints (Mormons), about 200 women reported problem pregnancies. A further examination of this group revealed that many of them were in fact not Mormon and the investigators were surprised to learn that thirteen of fourteen women who drank seven or more cups of coffee daily during their pregnancy reported miscarriages, foetal deaths, or stillbirths.

Adults are protected from potentially toxic effects of caffeine by rapidly metabolising it to less toxic metabolites: only 1 per cent of the original caffeine is excreted in the urine unchanged. The same does not occur in the neonate. When urine and plasma samples were taken from a hundred babies there was evidence that while drugs such as barbiturates crossed the placenta and were broken down to inactive compounds which were then excreted, caffeine remained largely unchanged. In neonatal tissues 75–83 per cent of ingested caffeine is excreted in the urine without being further metabolised. This also indicates that the foetus lacks the necessary caffeine-detoxifying enzymes.

Smoking has been associated with increased abortion rates, lowered birth rates and increased stillbirths. There are also increased incidences of antipartum haemorrhage, impaired brain development and possible teratogenic effects, all of which can be reversed if the mother gives up smoking during pregnancy. Data from the Royal Hospital for Women in Sydney has revealed that 21 per cent of smoking mothers have aborted at least once compared with 16 per cent for non-smokers. Stillbirths rose from 12 per 1,000 for non-smokers to 21 per 1,000 for those who smoked more than 10 cigarettes per day. A study of children from the British Perinatal Mortality Survey at the age of seven years found that children born of smoking mothers were smaller and slightly retarded in reading ability compared with contemporary children from non-smoking mothers. Experimental evidence from animals confirms that cigarette smoke does affect the brain. The offspring of rats exposed to cigarette smoke during pregnancy are found to have a reduction in the number of cells in various areas of the brain and hindbrain.

One of the most widely used drugs in our Western society is tetracycline. There is now documented evidence that it adversely affects birth weight and bone formation in the offspring of rats, mice, guinea pigs and chickens given the drug while they were pregnant. It has also been found in the bones of ten of twenty-three therapeutically aborted early foetuses taken from mothers who had received the drug in varying doses and for varying lengths of time. When taken in late pregnancy, tetracycline can adversely affect the deciduous teeth of the infant. Premature infants given tetracycline exhibit delayed bone growth, particularly of the fibula bone.

To some extent the foetus is protected from chemical exposure more than the lactating infant because it has the protection of the mother's liver and kidneys which help metabolise and excrete foreign chemicals before they gain entry to the placenta. On the other hand, drugs and other chemicals still have to traverse a complex barrier between the mother's blood and the breast milk which tends to result in lower levels of drugs in breast milk. The degree and rate at which a drug or chemical passes into breast milk depends upon several factors. The smaller water-soluble molecules pass into breast milk fairly easily while larger molecules have a much harder time gaining entry unless they are fat-soluble and as such can readily pass from the blood to the breast milk, tending to accumulate there.

Lactating women taking chloralhydrate or lithium have demonstrated breast milk levels of each drug at around 50 per cent of the blood level. Others, such as phenylbutazone, metranidazol (i.e. Flagyl) and chloramphenicol are excreted into breast milk at much lower levels, but have greater potential problems. Table 7.1 represents some of the most commonly prescribed drugs that are excreted into breast milk during lactation. Some of these drugs appear to be harmless while others should be avoided completely, or taken with caution after fully discussing the advantages and disadvantages with a medical practitioner.

Table 7.1   Safety of drugs excreted into breast milk

Drug	Excretion into breast milk	Safety
Alcohol	Milk levels are approximately equal to blood levels	Excessive drinking predisposes to Foetal Alcohol Syndrome (FAS); may inhibit oxytocin release and diminish milk secretion
Amantidine	Detectable, may cause adverse effects in infants	Use an alternative drug if possible
Aminophylline	Less than 1% excreted but is eliminated slowly, especially in premature infants	Sustained release preparations not recommended; feed just prior to taking the drug
Amitriptyline	Minimal amounts excreted	No reported harmful effects
Amoxycillin and Ampicillin	See penicillins	—
Antineoplastic Agents		Not recommended
Aspirin	Blood levels are higher than milk	Do not take high or prolonged doses
Atropine	Small amounts excreted; may diminish milk secretion	Caution with high doses

Table 7.1   (Cont'd)

Drug	Excretion into breast milk	Safety
Barbiturates	More excreted of the shorter acting drugs compared with the longer acting	Phenobarbitone may cause drowsiness; mothers should avoid single high doses
Caffeine	About 1% of oral dose is excreted	Infant irritability is reported at high doses; take 4–6 hours before feeding
Carbamazepine	Infant blood level the same as milk after 3 days	To be used with caution
β-Carotene	Present	Discolouration of infants skin is possible
Cephalosporins	Fairly low excretion rate	Not contra indicated
Chloral hydrate	Milk level is 50–80% of blood level	Causes drowsiness in infants at high doses
Chloramphenicol	Small amounts excreted	Avoid; potential bone marrow damage
Librium	Insignificant amounts	No recorded harmful effects
Chlormethiazole	Small amounts excreted	Not known
Chloroquine	Insignificant amounts excreted	Not known
Chlorthiazide	Very small amounts excreted	May diminish milk secretion in high doses
Chlorpromazine	Small amounts excreted	May cause sedation in infant
Cimetidine	Excreted	Not recommended
Codeine	Trace amounts	Not known
Corticosteroids	Excreted in small amounts	Not recommended in high doses or for long term usage
Dextropropoxy-phene	50% of blood level	Avoid in large or regular doses
Diazepam	Excretion varies	Metabolised slowly in infant; may cause jaundice; avoid
Diphenoxylate (Lomotil)	Not known	Not recommended
Ephedrine	Excreted	No known harmful effects
Ergot preparations	Excreted	Multiple doses postpartum suppress lactation; large doses contra-indicated
Erythromycin	Trace amounts	Not contra-indicated
Fluritrazepam	Trace amounts	Caution with high doses
Flurazepam	Trace amounts	Caution at high doses
Haloperidol	Small amounts	Use with caution only when essential
Imiprimine	Low levels	Use with caution
Indomethacin	Excreted	One report of convulsions in neonate
Iodides	Excreted	Contraindicated; affects thyroid function
Isoniazid	High levels in milk	Toxic to liver; contraindicated
Kanamycin	Small amounts	Not contraindicated
Lincomycin	Excreted	Not known
Lithium	33–50% of blood level	Not recommended
Marijuana	Low levels	Unknown

Table 7.1   (Cont'd)

Drug	Excretion into breast milk	Safety
Methadone	Small amounts	Caution with use
Metoprolol	Excreted	Unlikely to cause adverse effects
Metronidazole (Flagyl)	Excreted, mutagenic or carcinogenic potential	Withhold breast feeding for 12–24 hours after dose
Morphine	Excreted	Use low levels
Naproxen	1% of blood level	Avoid if possible
Nalidixic Acid	Small amounts	One report of haemolytic anaemia; caution if used
Nicotine	Excreted; may decrease milk supply and cause nausea and vomiting in infants	Smoking: avoid if possible
Oral contraceptives (includes oestrogens)	Small amounts	Combinations contraindicated; low dose progesterone products best suited during lactation
Paracetamol	Less than 0.1% of oral dose excreted	Not contraindicated
Penicillins	Small amounts	Caution with injectables
Phenylbutazone	Small amounts	Contraindicated; causes blood dyscrasias
Phenytoin	21% of blood level	Caution; adversely affects liver
Propranolol	Small amounts	Not contraindicated
Quinine	Small amounts	Potential risk of thrombocytopenia
Sulphasalazine	Small amounts	Treat with caution if necessary to use
Sulphonamides (in general)	Excreted	Contraindicated in G6PD deficiency; caution at other times
Tetracyclines	Variable excretion; absorption decreased by calcium in milk	Avoid; causes mottling in teeth
Theophylline	Less than 1% excreted; slowly metabolised	Feed just prior to drug intake
Thyroxine	Excreted in small amounts	Not contraindicated but may mask hypothyroid condition
Warfarin	Trace amounts	Infant may require vitamin K if in mother in large amounts

Source: Adapted from information supplied by Mr. Ron Batagol from the Drug Information Service, Royal Women's Hospital, Carlton, Victoria

8

Pesticide and herbicide residues in food

Coffs Harbour is a coastal town situated on the far north coast of New South Wales. Last year six children were born in the Coffs Harbour District Hospital with cleft palates, six times the national average, five within a few weeks of each other. In total, there were 21 congenital abnormalities reported out of 732 births during the year. These included shortened limbs and heart defects. In 1983 there were only three congenital abnormalities out of 727 births. In a nearby town, Bellingen, three babies were also born within three weeks of each other with a rare skull disorder called craniostenosis, a premature fusion of the bones of the skull. With this condition, unless surgery is undertaken, the child's brain outgrows the skull and brain damage occurs. It is usually so rare that you would not expect more than one occurrence per 10,000 births. However, suddenly there is a dramatic rise in this and other kinds of birth defects in this sleepy little coastal town — the banana capital of New South Wales.

Great interest has been shown by the media because in this same area hundreds of residents have suffered from gastrointestinal complaints characterised by severe diarrhoea, abdominal pain, vomiting, depression and lethargy. Mothers throughout the area have reported these same symptoms in their children, who are also suffering from impaired growth, sunken eyes and a bluey-grey look. Doctors, baffled at first, began treating patients with Flagyl, a drug used in the treatment of giardia and other parasitic infections of the intestinal tract. The Department of Health have been concerned that doctors were treating patients for giardia without any conclusive evidence of its existence, water tests for giardia and other parasites having come up negative. However, a public survey run by the local newspaper revealed that of the 566 families who replied, 331 complained of giardia-like symptoms.

Many of the 18-month-old infants born in the region weigh about the same as a 6-month-old and children 6 or 7 years of age have the growth of a 3-year-old. Some of these children have been taken to Sydney or Melbourne for specialist examination. Hospital tests, which have included barium meals, duodenal biopsies, blood screening and x-rays have again all come up negative. When some of the children were taken off their strong antibiotic and antiparasitic drugs, they immediately started to recover, some dramatically, until they returned to ·the Coffs Harbour area, where the symptoms immediately returned.

In the absence of any positive laboratory tests it is now suspected that chemical spraying of the area's banana crops may be responsible for many of these unsolved problems. Aerial and truck crop spraying are believed to contaminate both reservoir water and local crops. One of Coffs Harbour's main water reservoirs is situated in the middle of the banana plantations and planes have been seen spraying over it.

There are presently over twenty different types of chemicals registered for use on bananas in New South Wales and some of these, such as Fenaniphos, dimethoate 2, 4D and dieldrin have been banned overseas because of their potential danger and unpredictability. Early in 1985, 2, 4D and dieldrin were also banned in Australia, but farmers had stockpiled dieldrin and still regularly use it on their bananas. Other farmers have reportedly used much higher concentrations of the pesticides 'just to make sure'. Proper supervision of pesticide usage is nearly impossible. In New South Wales the Department of Agriculture has only one inspector to supervise the use of chemicals for the whole of the north coast region.

A number of stories about the positive association between illness and chemicals used for banana spraying has surfaced recently. The *Sydney Morning Herald* (16 October 1985) reported how a woman, Mrs. Simpson, and her four-year-old son were picking tomatoes from the family's garden at Boambee, ten kilometres south of Coffs Harbour: 'That morning, a truck in the area was spraying bananas for grubs and a fine spray of pesticide drifted over to blanket the family home.' Mrs. Simpson prepared tomatoes for lunch. 'As soon as they hit the stomach we were both violently ill,' she says. 'We were vomiting uncontrollably, our mouths were on fire, we didn't know what was happening to us.' Outside, the family's eight hens were lying on the ground. Four of them were found to be dead. The pet goat was also on the ground, and the next morning it gave birth eight weeks prematurely to two grossly deformed young.

The banana farmer had come over to the house and advised the Simpsons to vacate it for the day. 'He told me that he was supposed to use one part pesticide to ten parts of water but he was doing it the other way around to kill the grubs', Mrs. Simpson says.

Two weeks earlier, the family had suffered violent stomach cramps after a light plane had dumped chemicals over the house. The planes flew over daily during parts of the spraying season, from August to October, says Mrs. Simpson. 'The stuff would cling to your skin as if you'd sprayed yourself with something because the planes never shut off when they were flying over homes.'

Mrs. Simpson was continually ill up to the time when she gave birth to a still born baby girl in April 1982. During the pregnancy she was diagnosed as having giardia. She also had regular large boils on her eardrums. An autopsy on the baby showed her spine was deformed and some organs had failed to form. A year earlier, Mrs. Simpson had given birth to another still born baby girl with spina bifida and gross deformities to the head. Again, she had conceived during the spraying season. Mrs. Simpson's two other children, conceived before and after the family left the area, were both normal.

There are presently about 1,500 different chemicals in over 60,000 formulations which are available as synthetic organic pesticides. These include insecticides, herbicides, fungicides, nematicides, rodenticides and fumigants. They are systematically and seasonally sprayed, poured or dusted on cereals, fruit and vegetables before, during and after harvest. Many of these chemicals are also used on fallow land, cotton fields, grazing pastures, forests, golf courses and on building timber, woollen carpets, clothes and in our kitchens and pantries. Food contamination can arise due to spray drifting onto crops, solvents evaporating from timbers, carpets or clothes and aerosols in the home settling on exposed foods.

It is nearly impossible to avoid the effects of these chemicals in some form or another, though we can try to minimise our exposure to them. Edward Goldsmith, editor of the *Ecologist*, tells us that chemicals such as DDT have now become global contaminants. He says 'Traces are to be found in the bodies of Antarctic penguins, in the rain, in our drinking water, and in just about all commercially produced food. Each one of us has in his body fats, traces of hundreds of different pesticides. They are in human milk; they even find their way into fertilised eggs and contaminate foetuses in their mothers' wombs'. In Britain a report of the Food Additives and Contaminants Committee on Aldrin and Dieldrin Residues in Food says:

> We should like to recommend that no aldrin and dieldrin be permitted in milk and baby foods but we are aware that with the great sensitivity of analytical methods it has become possible to detect very low residues of aldrin and dieldrin in food and also that at present it would be impossible to produce milk or baby foods that were entirely free from aldrin and dieldrin. For these reasons we reluctantly decide against a zero tolerance and recommend that a limit of 0.003ppm be placed on aldrin and dieldrin in liquid milk, this being the lowest practicable limit of analysis. We recommend a corresponding limit of 0.02ppm in baby foods (including dried milk) which would take account of the difference in residues likely to be found in liquid and dried products. We also recommend that all ingredients for baby foods should be chosen by manufacturers with a view to keeping the aldrin and dieldrin content to the lowest possible level.
>
> (*Aldrin and Dieldrin in Food*, HMSO, 1967)

There are three major chemical groups of pesticides (insecticides). These are organochlorines, organophosphates and carbamates. A fourth category of synthetic pyrethroids such as permethrin, bioresmethrin, tetramethrin, allethrin, phenothrin, and deltamethrin are artificially synthesised compounds related to natural pyrethrins which are found in chrysanthemums.

Figure 8.1

Chemical structures of some organochlorines

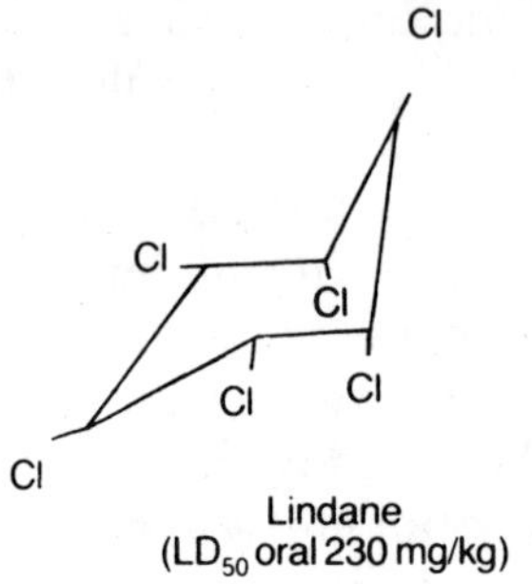

Lindane
(LD$_{50}$ oral 230 mg/kg)

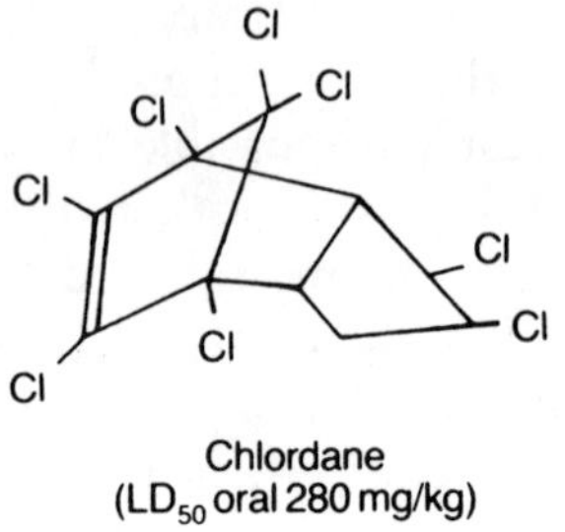

Chlordane
(LD$_{50}$ oral 280 mg/kg)

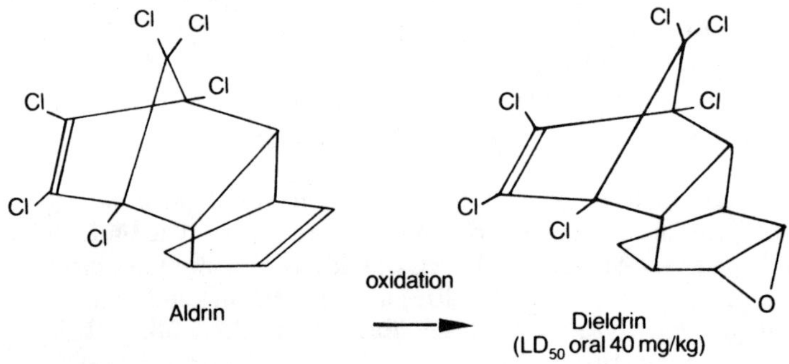

oxidation

Aldrin

Dieldrin
(LD$_{50}$ oral 40 mg/kg)

Lindane is the starting material used to make chlordane, aldrin, dieldrin, hep-tachlor and endrin. Lindane and chlordane are generally less toxic than aldrin which is less toxic than dieldrin. When absorbed into the body these pesticides are detoxified by the liver and excreted by the kidneys. Endrin has the shortest half life (the time it takes to reduce its concentration by 50%) – 3 hours, and it is also the most toxic. Dieldrin has a half life of 80 days and DDT 100 days. Small amounts of these pesticides are stored in body fat and are released during periods of stress or ill health.

These substances have generally low toxicity in mammals including humans and are biodegradable, with the exception of deltamethrin.

Organochlorines such as chlordane, DDT, lindane and aldrin are highly toxic, and are not biodegradable. They last for de-cades in the soil and being fat soluble, can be stored in human fat tissues, liver and the central nervous system to produce suspected chronic and delayed effects. Organochlorines are heavily restricted in many industrialised nations, and in 1985 were restricted for some purposes in Australia. Voluntary limitation of the use of dieldrin and aldrin came into effect in Britain in 1965 but studies on the eggs of sparrowhawks in fourteen different areas around the country during 1971–77 showed no decline in organochlorine residues, and in some cases there has been evidence of an increase. This indicates that the use of these substances is more extensive than generally admitted, or they are not used according to instructions or, perhaps, that their persistence in the food and animal chain is longer than estimated.

A more likely explanation is the fact that dieldrin and aldrin

Table 8.1   Common organochlorine pesticides and herbicides

Chemical name	Trade name	Use and toxic effects
Dicamba	Banex Banair	Herbicide, toxic at low concentrations to non-target plants
MCPA	Methoxone	Weed killer, extremely toxic to non-target plants
Pentachlorophenol	PCP	Herbicide, carcinogenic in animal tests, toxic to bees
Picloram	Tordon	Herbicide, non-biodegradable
Sodium trichloroacetate	TCA	Herbicide, toxic to worms at normal concentration, corrosive to skin
2,4-D	Multiple names including Amine 50 Amidox 50 Dacamime 4-D Lane Delamex Weed Killer	Destroys broad leafed leaves in cereal crops; foetotoxic, carcinogenic, teratogenic; must not be used near water bodies
2,4,5,-T	Multiple names including Ban-Oxalis Tordon 105 tree Killer Weedone Shell herbicide B80	Woody weed killer especially blackberries, used extensively by sugar cane growers and government authorities Foetotoxic, teratogenic, carcinogenic Must not be used near water bodies
Aldrin	Aldrex	Insecticide used for termite control; accumulates in body, toxic to fish and birds

138

Table 8.1   (Cont'd)

Chemical name	Trade name	Use and toxic effects
Chlordane	Chlordane	Insecticide used for domestic pest control, used on citrus fruits in some states; Banned in United States in 1982, being suspected of causing cancer in humans
DDT	DDT	Insecticide, present in all living things, non-biodegradable; suspected carcinogen; toxic to bird life; still has limited use on some food crops in Australia
Dieldrin	Dieldrin	See Aldrin
Endrin	Endrin	Insecticide, accumulates in body; suspected carcinogen. Most uses cancelled in United States by 1979
Endosulfan	Endopest Thiodan	Insecticide for use on vegetables and cereal crops; extreme toxicity to fish and wildlife
Heptachlor	Heptachlor	Pest control in buildings and housing; Phased out in United States by 1982; suspected carcinogen
Lindane	Grammexane	Vegetable crops and against fleas, mites and wood boring insects; highly toxic central nervous system stimulant

are still allowed in Britain for use in certain circumstances on winter sown wheat, sugar beet seed, potatoes, brassicas, hop roots, barley, bean, onion and strawberry seeds and spinach. However there is no way of monitoring the uses of these insecticides.

In Australia, aldrin is still in limited use for timber treatment to control termites, and on citrus fruits, even though it is considered a human carcinogen by the United States Environmental Protection Authority and residues may remain for up to seventeen years. Aldrin has been used in the past as a soil insecticide in sugar cane production in Australia with no requirements for a maximum residue limit.

Organochlorines have also found their way into the upper

atmosphere over the last few decades. There are 20,000 tons of polychlorinated biphenyls in the upper 200 metres of the North Atlantic and American white-tailed eagles carry approximately 14,000ppm. A survey carried out on the remote Enewetak Atoll in the North Pacific Ocean has also demonstrated measurable amounts of lindane, chlordane and dieldrin in both air and rain water. Closer to our main areas of civilisation we find hepta-chlor (a very toxic metabolite of chlordane) in the fat tissue of 96 per cent of the population. Heptachlor epoxide and dieldrin residues are found in 88 per cent of a population sample in Ottawa, Canada, and 96 per cent in Kingston, Jamaica. The body fat tissue of Australians is known to contain 2½ times the dieldrin content (0.67ppm) of subjects selected from 10 other countries. This is because Australia has continued to use organochlorines when other countries have restricted their use, especially during the 1960s and 1970s. Though it should be pointed out that even though Iraq banned aldrin and dieldrin in 1976 and has never used heptachlor, its average level of dieldrin in lamb fat in 1985 was 0.067ppm and in beef fat 0.101ppm. Chlordane and heptachlor and their residues amount to 0.193ppm in lamb and beef fat. This situation reflects the increasing burden of organochlorines in the biosphere.

Organochlorines become most hazardous to human health through a process called biomagnification. Spray drifts and drain-offs from treated fields contaminate water bodies. Small plankton and other organisms living in the water absorb the pesticides and start to accumulate them in their tissues. The next animal in the food chain, feeding on the plankton, takes in a diet enriched with the pesticide residues and their metabolites. After a period of time the concentration of these residues rises in the animal and there is a stepwise increase in pesticide concen-tration along the food chain.

A good example of this ecological magnification of organo-chlorines is demonstrated in the case of contamination of Clear Lake, California with 0.02ppm DDD (the DDT metabolite). The concentration in plankton rose to 5.3ppm (×265), small fish 10.0ppm, predatory fish 1,700ppm (×85,000) and preda-tory birds 1,600ppm (×80,000). Five years after the initial con-tamination of the lake there was an increase in mortality in carnivorous birds, and predatory fish were found to contain

2,000ppm of the insecticide. One study on fish has revealed that chlordane becomes bioconcentrated about 10,000 times, a sobering thought for those eating fish from harbours and estuaries where the population density is greatest or which take in polluted rivers.

The ecological magnification of dieldrin fed to rats at 50ppm results in a blood level of 0.047ppm, the liver 1.01ppm and fat 6.42ppm within 24 hours. After 31 days of dieldrin feeding the blood levels rise to 0.236ppm, the liver 12.70 (magnification ×53) and fat 280ppm (magnification ×1,182).

Such results give a clear demonstration that blood and urine levels of organochlorines do not accurately reflect the real body burden. It is not surprising to learn that the organochlorine compounds hexachlorohexane, DDT, hexachlorobenzene and polychlorinated biphenyls (PCBs) all accumulate in human adipose tissue with increasing age.

Pacific oysters taken from nineteen different sites in Tasmania have been found to contain up to 0.39ppm, the source of contamination thought to be an industrialised factory which used dieldrin to treat woollen fabrics. But of all the animals, birds appear to be affected most adversely by organochlorines, possibly because they are at the end of the food chain. Migratory birds from Tasmania and some small islands off the Australian coastline contain 18ppm dieldrin and 9ppm lindane. Forktailed kites from Alice Springs contain 10ppm in their body fat. Australian pelicans have been found with 5–10ppm and kookaburras with up to 1,058ppm. Marsupials such as the platypus, kangaroo and wallaby are particularly at risk because these animals have a prolonged suckling period and tend to concentrate fat-soluble organochlorine residues in their milk.

Since 1981 The Toxic and Hazardous Chemicals Committee of the Total Environment Centre in Sydney has been collecting evidence that organochlorine pesticides are being misused in both agriculture, especially the dairy industry, and in the urban pest control industry where firms have continually used chemicals without permits. Current legitimate urban uses of aldrin, dieldrin, heptachlor and chlordane in New South Wales, according to schedules published in May 1985, include applications to control the following pests — termites, borers, spiders, ants, cockroaches, silverfish, fleas, centipedes, beetles,

Figure 8.2   Chemical structures of some additional organochlorines

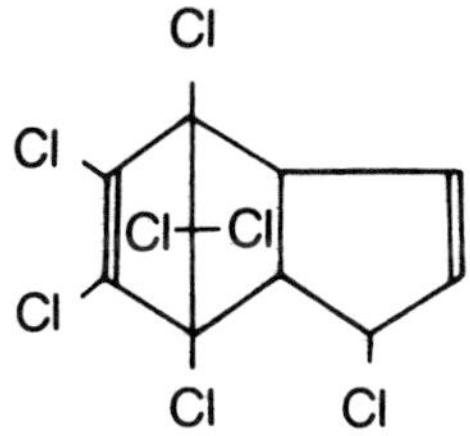

Heptachlor

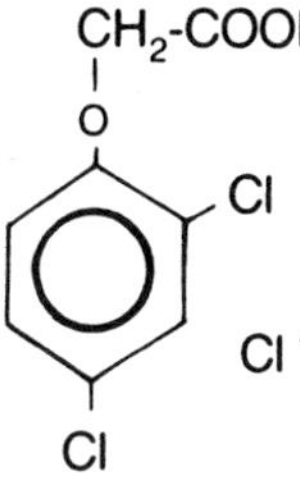

2,4 D

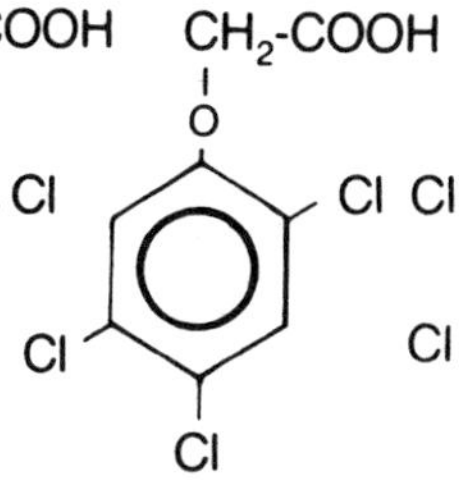

2,4,5 T

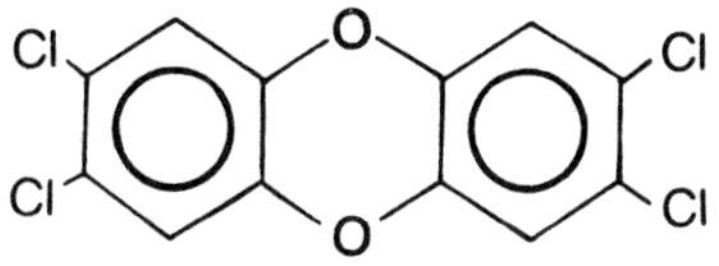

TCDD
(Tetrachlorodibenzo-p-dioxin)
(Dioxin)

Polychlorinated bipnenyls

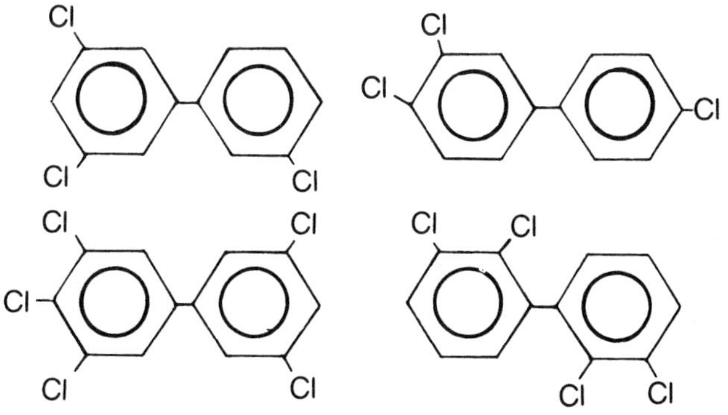

142

Figure 8.3   Degradation products of DDT

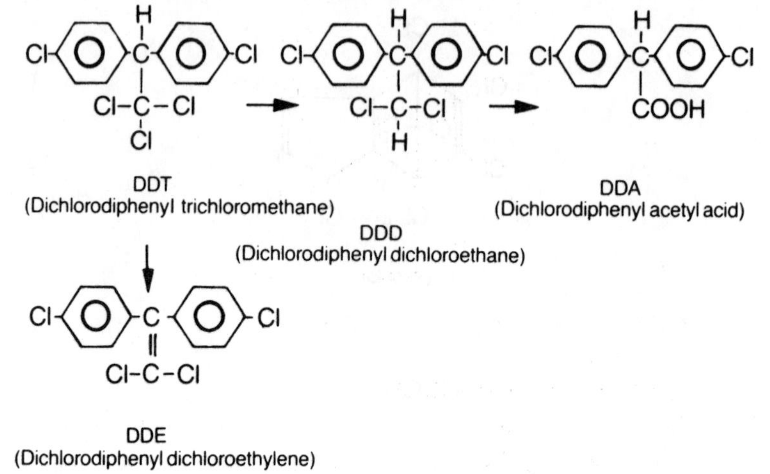

DDT
(Dichlorodiphenyl trichloromethane)

DDA
(Dichlorodiphenyl acetyl acid)

DDD
(Dichlorodiphenyl dichloroethane)

DDE
(Dichlorodiphenyl dichloroethylene)

grubs, crickets, earwigs, slaters, cutworms, weevils and wireworms. Allowable applications are limited to subfloor areas, eaves, outside walls and paths but not to interior living areas. Lindane may be used for the control of bed bugs, fleas, flies, honey bees, mosquitoes, moths, spiders, beetles and paper wasps. Lindane smoke generators are readily available in chemists, hardware stores and nurseries. Contamination of air, land, water and food from spray drift, surface accumulation and run off may be significant as there are no guarantees of safety, or tight controls on usage. While urban usage has not been restricted the new schedules of the Pesticides Act published in May 1985 have banned all organochlorines for agricultural use in New South Wales, with the exception of DDT for the control of pests in stone and pomme fruit.

In the past, agricultural practices in New South Wales have included the use of organochlorine pesticides to control the proliferation of insects affecting cereal crops, maize, sugar, bananas, carrots, potatoes, stone fruits, pomme fruits and other staples, including crops and pastures used for animal feed. The residues from these pesticides have accumulated in the soil and subsequently have found their way into cattle, resulting in the quarantining of some animals. This same problem is now also

Figure 8.4

Dieldrin contaminates cow's milk
The pesticides dieldrin and heptachlor have been found in cow's milk in six different localities around New South Wales. The supply of milk from dairy farms in Kempsey, Wauchope, Gloucester, Dungog, Singleton, Hexham and Bodalla (a major cheese making centre on the south coast) was suspended recently when the dieldrin concentration was found to be 10–100 times the highest acceptable level set by the National Health and Medical Research Council. The problem appears to have arisen because of either illegal spraying of stockfeed or contamination of feed grown in soils contaminated with soil residues. Dieldrin and other organochlorines have a half-life in the soil of twelve to fifteen years.

facing the sugar cane industry since the world market downturn in sales has put many cane growers out of business. Because their land is so contaminated with residues they are unable to grow alternative food crops, which are free of contamination.

Presently in the state of Victoria, aldrin and dieldrin have been approved for limited agricultural uses: the control of termites, argentine ants and black beetle. It can still be used in the home garden, for general horticulture, in farm, industrial and public health situations and for various pests. Chlordane has no proclaimed approved uses and heptachlor can be used for termite control and the control of insects in hides and skins.

Early in 1985, New York state issued an emergency ban on all uses of chlordane, aldrin and dieldrin. Present restrictions on uses of aldrin, dieldrin, chlordane and heptachlor in other countries are shown in Table 8.2.

Organophosphates are another major group of pesticides (insecticides) which act by blocking nerve transmission in the insect by inhibiting a vital enzyme called cholinesterase. Examples include dichlorovos (DDVP), maldison (Malathion), diazinon and chlorpyrifos. These substances are often highly toxic and, being volatile, can be easily inhaled. They are more biodegradable than the organochlorines, but are still suspected of chronic and delayed effects — especially with dichlorovos.

Carbamates have the same mode of action (i.e. as nerve poisons) as the organophosphates, but their toxicities are variable. The most toxic carbamate is carbaryl which is thought

Table 8.2 Worldwide restrictions on uses of common organochlorine pesticides now banned in the United States

	Aldrin	Dieldrin	Chlordane	Heptachlor
EEC	Prohibited except for special soil treatment	Prohibited for marketing	Prohibited for marketing	Prohibited for marketing
Canada	Registered for termite control	Termite control only	Restricted for soil and structural insects	Banned except for flower bulbs
Finland	Banned except for use on export particle boards	Heavily restricted	Banned	Restricted for some timber products
Israel	Banned	Banned	Approved for use only as bait	Approved for use only in treatment of soil
Hungary	Banned	Banned	Banned	Banned
Cyprus	Banned for agricultural use	Banned for agricultural use	Banned for agricultural use	Banned for agricultural use
Japan	Prohibited except by authorisation of cabinet	Banned	Banned	Banned
NZ	Permit required	Commercial use only; permit required	25% or more in a product must be labelled 'poison'; Permit required	Voluntarily withdrawn from market
Norway	Registration withdrawn	Registration withdrawn	New registrations banned	—
Sweden	Prohibited except by permit	Banned	Withdrawn from domestic use; no longer manufactured	Not approved for use as pesticide
Turkey	Banned	Banned	Banned	Banned

Figure 8.5

Chemical structures of some organophosphate pesticides

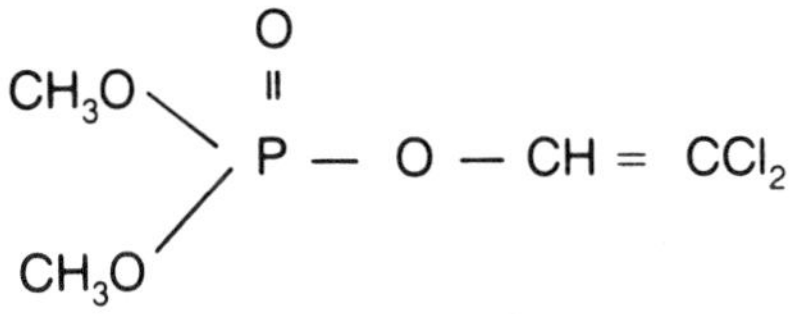

$$CH_3O$$
$$CH_3O$$
$$P - O - CH = CCl_2$$

Dichlorvos (Shelltox strips)

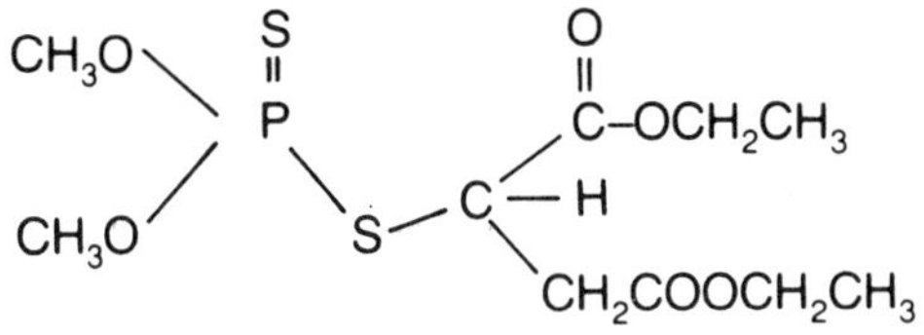

Maldison (Malathion)

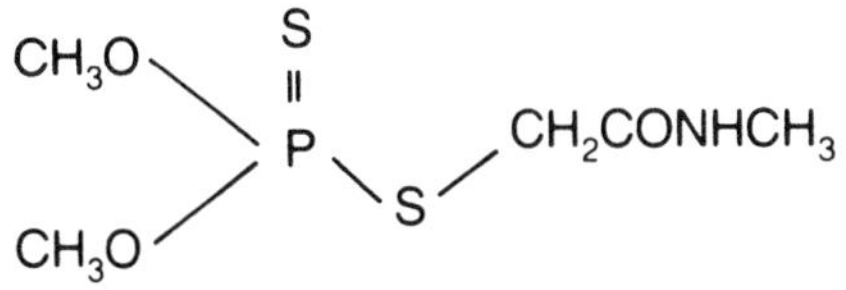

Dimethoate (Rogor)

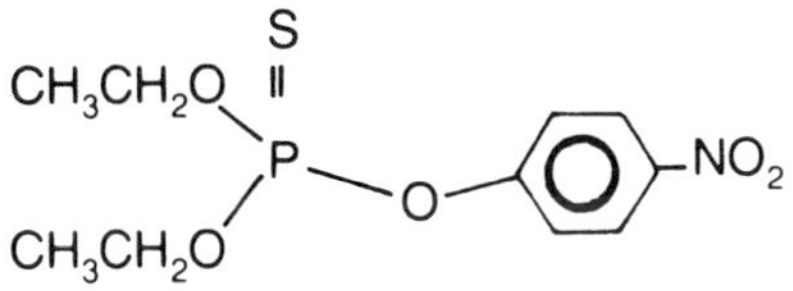

Parathion

Parathion has a half life of 4 months and has been responsible for more acciden-tal deaths than any other pesticide (LD_{50} oral/rat 10mg/kg). While maldison has a similar half life it has a much lower toxicity for mammals (LD_{50} oral/rat 1,300 mg/kg) because in man and other mammals (but not in insects) it is easily detoxified to a water soluble substance which is then excreted. Dichlorovos is continuously emitted from Shelltox strips to saturate the domestic atmosphere. While it has a half life of only 8 hours it is still quite toxic to mammals (LD_{50} oral/rat 30mg/kg) and should never be used in any areas of a house (or restaurant) where food is being stored, prepared or served.

to be converted into a potent carcinogen in the stomach and may cause sterility. Other examples include propoxur, bendiocarb, methiocarb, and captan.

A few highly toxic and persistent inorganic insecticides are also presently marketed in Australia and these include arsenic, boron, sodium fluoride and sodium cyanide.

The major herbicides are also organochlorines (2,4-D, 2,4,5,-T, MCPA, PCP Picloram, Dicamba and sodium trichloroacetate) but include others such as paraquat, diquat, MSMA, simazine, amitrole, DSMA and glycerophosphate.

Rodenticides used to control rats and mice include warfarin, thallium sulphate, bromadiolone and coumatretralyl. Molluscides used to control slugs and snails include methioncarb (carbamate). Fungicides include pentachorophenol, copper arsenate, Benomyl, cadmium chloride, captan, Maneb, Mancozeb, Thiram and Zineb and a fumigant commonly used in Australia, ethylene dibromide, recommended for use by bee keepers.

Over twenty years ago in Britain a survey of the levels of pesticides (above reporting levels) in different foods sampled revealed residues of organochlorine pesticides in: 41 per cent of

Table 8.3   Common organophosphate pesticides

Chemical name	Trade name	Use and toxicity
Demeton-S-methyl	Metasystox	Insecticide, toxic to bees at normal concentrations
Dichlorovos	Shelltox strips Nuvan Mafu	Insecticides, mutagen in test animals
Diazinon	Diazamin Basudin Gesapon	Sheep dip; must not be used near water bodies
Dimethoate	Rogor	Insecticide; banned in United States in 1981; risk of carcinogenic, mutagenic and foetogenic properties
Disulfoton	Disyston	Insecticide; restricted in United States in 1979; high skin and lung toxicity
Fenthion	Lebaycid Baytex	Insecticide; highly toxic to domestic animals, poultry, birds and bees
Maldison	Malathion	Insecticide; toxic to bees
Naled	Dibrom	Insecticide; highly corrosive to skin and toxic to bees
Parathion	Folidol E605	Insecticide; restricted in United States; toxic to skin and lungs

hard cheeses, 28 per cent of soft cheeses, 45 per cent of butter, 33 per cent of infant food and 65 per cent of strawberries. Organophosphate residues above reporting levels were also found in 17 per cent of strawberries, 11 per cent of peaches, 10 per cent of grapefruit, and carbamates in 47 per cent of eggs, 39 per cent of hard cheeses and 35 per cent of soft cheeses. Since this time there has been a sharp rise in the use of both herbicides and insecticides containing these substances.

There is a wealth of information on acute toxicity and toxicity arising from accidental sprayings and accidental poisonings, but as with the case of synthetic food additives, the adequacy of testing of pesticides is highly questionable. Carcinogenic effects take twenty to thirty years to appear after exposure to the carcinogen. Mutagenic effects can surface generations after the initial exposure. Nor has the possible adverse effect of pesticide residues on behaviour been examined. There has been surprisingly little work carried out to examine the possible adverse interactions between different pesticides,

Figure 8.6

Organochlorines attack health

The United States National Cancer Institute in a classification of carcinogens in drinking water lists aldrin, chlordane, heptachlor, heptachlor epoxide and lindane as suspected carcinogens and dieldrin as a recognised carcinogen.

(Source: Kraybill, M.F., Environmental Science Health C1, 175–8, 1983)

A group of women who had premature deliveries had serum levels of heptachlor-epoxide and other organochlorines signifiantly higher (200 per cent) than the organochlorine concentrations in serum of normal third trimester women.

(Source: Wasserman, M. *et al.*, *Annals of the New York Academy of Science* 320, 69–124, 1979)

Rare neuroblastoma tumours have been reported in five children exposed to chlordane, either *in utero* or in early childhood. Also three cases of acute leukaemia and three cases of aplastic leukaemia have been reported in adults who had been exposed to chlordane.

(Infante, P.F., *et al. Scandinavian Journal of Work, Environment and Health* 4, 137–50 1978)

and between pesticides and other compounds used during crop production. The cumulative effect of chronic low–dose exposure of a single pesticide and the additive effect of small quantities of many different pesticides have also not been examined.

The control of pesticide usage in Australia, Britain and the United States is not only extremely difficult but is based on the mistaken premise that there is a fixed 'safe level'. However, this level for a foetus and infant may be different from that of an adult. Individuals with liver or kidney disease have 100 to 1000 times greater sensitivity to these substances compared with a healthy person because their ability to detoxify and elimiante small quantities of ingested chemicals is dramatically reduced. In this respect many fat–soluble environmental pollutants from industry, as well as agriculture, such as polychlorinated biphenyls (PCBs) are regularly found in breast milk, with their effect on the infant still not known.

In an attempt to control the level of pesticide residues in Australia the Commonwealth Department of Health has published a book entitled *Standard for Maximum Residue Limits of Pesticides, Agricultural Chemicals, Food Additives, Veterinary Medicines and Noxious Substances in Food.* Examples of the maximum limits for major herbicides, insecticides, rodenticides, fumigants and fungicides are shown in Table 8.4. Most of the values are arbitrarily chosen at or about the limit of analytical detection

Table 8.4   **Maximum residue limits of some Australian pesticides presently used in association with the production of the food concerned (limit set at or about the limit of analytical determination)**

Substance	Maximum residue limit (mg/kg)	Food
Aldrin (dieldrin)	0.2	Fat of meat
	0.15	Milk and milk products (fat basis), goat milk (fat basis)
	0.1	Eggs (shell free), asparagus, cole crops, carrots, cucumber, eggplant, horse-radish, lettuce, onions, parsnips, peppers, pimentos, potatoes, radishes and radish tops
	0.05	Citrus fruit
	0.001	Water

Table 8.4   (Cont'd)

Substance	Maximum residue limit (mg/kg)	Food
Chlordane (sum of cis and trans chlordane and oxychlordane)	0.5	Crude linseed oil, crude soybean oil
	0.3	Sugar beet
	0.1	Crude cottonseed oil, cucurbits, pineapples
	0.05	Cereal grain, milk and milk products (fat basis), fat of meat
	0.02	Vegetables (except cucurbits), eggs, citrus, stone and pomme fruits, edible cottonseed oil, edible soy bean oil
	0.006	Water
DDT (including DDD and DDE)	7.0	Fat of meat of cattle, sheep, pigs, goats and poultry, leafy vegetables
	3.0	Fruit (other than citrus)
	1.25	Milk and milk products (fat basis) goat milk (fat basis)
	1.0	Edible oils, fish, seed and pod vegetables, margarine, root vegetables, tomatoes
	0.5	All other vegetables, eggs
	0.2	Citrus fruit
	0.1	Cereal grains
	0.003	Water
2,4D	5.0	Citrus, sugar cane
	2.0	Edible offal of cattle, pigs, sheep and goats
	0.2	Meat, cereal grains
	0.1	Potatoes, water
Dimethoate	5.0	Strawberries (witholding period one day)
	2.0	Vegetables (except tomatoes and peppers), fruits (except strawberries)
	1.0	Tomatoes and peppers
Heptachlor (including its epoxide)	0.5	Crude soybean oil
	0.2	Fat of meat, carrots
	0.15	Milk and milk products (fat basis)
	0.05	Vegetables (except carrots and tomatoes), eggs
	0.02	Cereal grains, tomatoes, cotton seed, soy beans, edible soy bean oil
	0.01	Pineapple, citrus fruit
	0.003	Water
Lindane	3.0	Cherries, cranberries, grapes, plums, strawberries
	2.0	Fat of meat of cattle, goats, sheep and pigs, vegetables, all other fruit

Table 8.4 **(Cont'd)**

Substance	Maximum residue limit (mg/kg)	Food
	1.0	Fish
	0.7	Poultry (fat basis)
	0.5	Cereal grains
	0.2	Milk and milk products (fat basis), goat milk (fat basis)
	0.1	Eggs, egg pulp, water
	0.05	Oil seeds
Maldison	20.0	Wheat bran
	8.0	Cereal grains, dried fruit, nuts, dried beans, lentils, peanuts
	4.0	Citrus fruit
	3.0	Tomatoes, kale
	2.0	Most fruit, vegetables and whole meal flour from wheat and rye
	1.0	Strawberries, fat of meat, all poultry, eggs, milk and milk products (fat basis)
	0.5	Pears, blueberries, peas, cauliflowers, collard peppers, eggplant, kohlrabi, root vegetables, Swiss chard, turnip
	0.1	Water
Paraquat	10.0	Rice (in husk)
	1.0	Olives (fresh)
	0.5	Rice (polished), sorghum, edible offal
	0.2	Cottonseed, potatoes, dried hops
	0.1	Maize, soybeans
	0.05	Other vegetables, fruit, sugar cane, nuts, cereal grains (other than rice and maize), meat
	0.04	Water
Parathion	1.0	Peaches, apricots, cottonseed
	0.7	Vegetables (except carrots)
	0.5	All other fruits, cereal grains, carrots, cottonseed oil
	0.03	Water

Note: A complete list of the maximum residue limits of pesticides, agricultural chemicals, feed additives, veterinary medicines and noxious substances in food is available in the Commonwealth Department of Health publication entitled *Standard for Maximum Residue Limits of Pesticides, Agricultural Chemicals, Feed Additives, Veterinary Medicines and Noxious Substances in Food*, Australian Government Publishing Service, Canberra, 1985.

and levels at or below this limit are considered to pose no threat to human health when foods containing these chemicals are ingested. Some of the substances which are exempted from the requirements of a maximum residue limit are also shown in Table 8.5.

Table 8.5   Substances which are exempted from the requirements of a maximum residue limit in Australia

Chemical name	Use
Aldrin	Timber treatment; soil insecticide in sugar cane production
Bacillus toyoi	Growth promotant in pigs and cattle
Benzalkonium chloride	For use as a teat dip
Chlordane	Timber treatment
Chlorflurenol	Growth regulator in pineapples
Creosote	Timber treatment, treatment for tree trunks and poultry houses
2,4-D	Herbicide on pastures
DDT	Insecticide on linseed; treatment of seed rice
Ethylene	Ripening of fruit
Formaldehyde	Seed dressing; fumigant of seed beds and animal houses
Formalin	Soil fumigant
Gonadotrophin	Induction of super ovulation in cattle, pigs and sheep
Heptachlor	Timber treatment
Lindane	Locust control on pastures; seed dressing; insecticide in sugar cane production
Methiocarb	Bait for the control of garden pests
Oestradiol benzoate	In combination with progesterone, in an intravaginal device for the regulation of oestrus in cattle When implanted in the ear for growth promotion purposes in cattle
Oestradiol-17-beta	When implanted in the ear for growth promotion purposes in cattle
Paraquat	Herbicide on pastures
Progesterone	Induction of oestrus in sheep, cattle and goats When implanted in the ear for growth promotion in cattle
Prostianol	Oestrus control in cattle and sheep
Strychnine	Rodenticide
2,4,5-T	Herbicide on pastures and sugar cane, fruit-setting spray for apricots; herbicide for control of blackberries
Testosterone cypionate	Growth promotant in sheep when injected subcutaneously
Testosterone enanthate or propionate	Control of posthitis and balanitis in sheep

* These substances are deemed unlikely to produce residues in food when used in accordance with good agricultural practice and when used as directed; any residues which may result from such use are not regarded as a hazard to human health.

Note: A complete list is available in *Standards for Maximum Residue Limits of Pesticides, Agricultural Chemicals, Feed Additives, Veterinary Medicines and Noxious Substances in Food* Australian Government Publishing Service. Canberra (1985) — ISBN 0 644 03856 X

One of the problems with having residue limits of pesticides and other chemicals is the appropriate action that should be taken if crops or a particular food suddenly exceeds the maximum residue level. There was a good example of this recently in the United States. There, the Food and Drug

Administration is supposed to set tolerance levels for environmental food contaminants which can't be entirely avoided. But the FDA has only set one such limit, in 1973, on polychlorinated biphenyls. Instead it adopts what it calls 'action levels' which it has done for more than twenty different contaminants ranging from lead and methanol to herbicides and pesticides. 'Action levels' simply means that if a manufacturer has toxins below these then they are legally within the limit, and the FDA cannot prosecute. Recently corn growers in South Carolina had a very dry summer, causing an increase in aflatoxins in the corn. Whereas normally the FDA action level was 20 parts per billion, the growers found that the level of aflatoxin far exceeded this. The FDA wrote a letter lifting the action level, allowing the growers to sell grain at 300 parts per billion. When the consumer group Public Citizen founded by Ralph Nader heard about this they sued the FDA which has since argued that fixed tolerance limits are too inflexible, and also that they don't have the resources to work out tolerances for all environmental contaminants. The fact that the FDA is now studying the feasibility of permanently raising the action levels to 300 parts per billion for aflatoxin (when we consider in Britain and Australia that the legal limit is still 10–15 parts per billion), really makes a mockery of the concept of maximum residue limits, tolerance levels or even action levels. Obviously the criteria for these limitations or tolerance levels must revolve entirely around public health factors and safety if consumers are to be protected.

It is disconcerting to discover that chemical pesticides and herbicides that are still freely available in one country have been banned in another because of fears of carcinogenicity and teratogenicity, quite apart from potential problems with chemical hypersensitivity arising from residues in food. The following substances have either been banned completely, phased out or their uses severely restricted in the United States over the last ten years: paraquat, parathion, lindane, DDT, dimethoate (dust formulation), dieldrin (aldrin), chlordane, heptachlor, 2,4,5-T, mirex, disulfoton, endrin, DBCP and mercury. More information on these bans or restrictions can be found in *Suspended and Cancelled Pesticides*, a publication of the United States Environmental Protection Agency (EPA), October 1979.

A more conservative approach would certainly seem justified in the light of the new scientific evidence surfacing each year. Recently scientists have found that dioxins (polychlorinated agents which arise from smoke-stacks of municipal waste incinerators burning plastics and also a contaminant of 2,4,5-T) are stored in the human body for longer than in animals. The half life in humans is about five years. This finding indicates that previous acceptable daily intakes will have to be reduced. Background levels of dioxin in the fat tissue of most people

Figure 8.7

Birth defects and the use of herbicides in Australia

In the 1970s in Australia there appears to have been a very highly significant increase in neonatal deaths (death in the first 28 days of life) from the congenital defects spina bifida (an 84% increase in deaths) and urinary system abnormalities, especially renal agenesis or imperfect kidney development (97% increase). Both kinds of defect have been reported elsewhere to be connected statistically with the chemical TCDD, an impurity of 2,4,5-T, which is a herbicide widely used in Australia in the late 60s and early 70s. 2,4,5-T is a major component of the defoliant Agent Orange. Late in the 1960s large quantities of this defoliant which contained levels of TCDD considered dangerously high were removed from Vietnam after fears were expressed about its foetal toxicity and teratogenicity. Some of it may have entered the world market, and it is possible that it reached Australia via Singapore between 1968 and 1971, although information on the precise nature of chemicals of this type entering Australia at this time has not been disclosed by the government.

P. Hall, from the Department of Statistics, and B. Selinger from the Department of Chemistry, Australian National University, Canberra, Australia have suggested that there may be a link between the abnormally high (they term it 'epidemic') proportions of the birth defects outlined above and the widespread use of defoliants containing TCDD in Australia. Because TCDD may remain in the body for a long term, even very low levels of exposure to this chemical could result in a substantial build-up in the population with the risk of a continuing high level of birth abnormalities. In addition, the expensive government funded study of the effects of Agent Orange on Vietnam veterans, which presumes no TCDD exposure for those who were not in Vietnam, would obviously be faced with some difficulties in interpretation of its results.

(Chemistry in Australia 48, 131–2, 1981)

living in Europe, Japan, Canada and the United States are about the same.

The dioxin ADI (acceptable daily intake) set for these countries based on animal toxicity studies is 1–10 picograms per kilogram of body weight per day. However, the new human half life figure for dioxins suggests that an ADI of at most 0.1 picograms (0.1×10^{-12} grams) would be more acceptable. This is highly significant when we realise that most people are presently getting around 3–16 picograms per kg per day. While this may not seem like such a large amount it could certainly cause problems for people with specific chemical sensitivities. McGovern found that three quarters of hyperactive children were exquisitely sensitive to just trace amounts of hydrocarbons, petrol, diesel fumes, outgassing paints, formaldehyde, aerosols and phenolic substances. Another researcher, William Rea, has also showed that patients with thrombophlebitis (an inflammatory disease of the blood vessels) became completely free of their symptoms when they were maintained in a special chemical free environment where foods, air and water were strictly monitored. Five out of ten of these symptom free patients contracted phlebitis again when challenged with only 0.0134ppm of the pesticide 2,4 DNP. Many also reacted to phenol (0.0024ppm), formaldehyde (0.2ppm) and petroleum alcohol (0.5ppm). It is accepted that chlorine in

Figure 8.8

Chemical to make ripening apples redder is questioned
The United States Environment Protection Agency (EPA) has recently issued a draft notice of its intention to ban the growth inhibitor Alar (daminozide) which is currently sprayed on young apple trees in the United States and Australia to limit their growth and allow more trees to be planted. It is also sprayed on ripening apples to make them redder. The EPA's current review of this product has uncovered research showing it to cause cancerous tumours in laboratory animals. Low levels of the substance have been found in apple juice and apple sauce according to chemists from Gerber Products, the largest American manufacturer of baby food. When Alar is heated during the processing of food it forms another substance (ultradimethyl hydrazine) which may be an even more potent carcinogen than the parent chemical.

drinking water is safe for human consumption at about 1.0ppm. Fifty per cent of the phlebitis patients, however, found that their symptoms were triggered at less than 0.33ppm and were even troubled by fumes from their shower, bath or dishwater.

Many individuals are already sensitive to small quantities of chemicals in our environment. Over the next few years it would not be at all surprising to find that the trace quantities of pesticides and herbicides that find their way into our daily food supply constitute a major source of adverse food chemical sensitivity reactions.

9

Naturally occurring food drugs and toxins

Many foods contain naturally occurring chemicals which act on the body in the same way as drugs to cause what is called a pharmacological effect. This occurs when a chemical agent such as a drug, hormone or related chemical messenger acts on a specialised part of a cell called a receptor site. In this way the action of tissues or organs can be externally controlled. Modern day drugs are usually analogues of naturally occurring hormones and neurotransmitters. When a drug binds to a receptor site it relays signals to the inside of the cell telling it how to behave and controls its metabolism. For example, the bronchodilator drug Ventalin, used by asthmatics, binds to receptor sites on the bronchial smooth muscle cells in the lungs, and signals them to relax. This command results in bronchodilatation, with the relaxed muscles inside the air tubes allowing a free passage of air into the lungs. Another substance, histamine, acts in the reverse way and on different receptors to cause bronchoconstriction by contracting the smooth muscle cells of the bronchial tubes.

In this way modern drug research has produced agents which can predictably reduce intestinal activity, block nerve impulses, increase and decrease heart rate and blood pressure, dilate or constrict blood vessels and virtually control most of the biological functions in the body. A vast array of modern pharmaceutical agents is now effectively used to ameliorate signs and symptoms associated with most clinical disorders simply by

156

manipulating the physiological and metabolic processes which mediate the functions.

When foods contain compounds which are chemically related to these drugs, hormones and neurotransmitters, they can cause the same type of reaction as if the drug itself had been taken. The most common naturally occurring 'drugs' in foods are the biologically active amines.

These are low-molecular weight substances which arise naturally as a consequence of metabolic processes in animals, plants and microorganisms. Most of them are derived from amino acids or related aromatic amino compounds and are structurally similar to hormones in our body, such as adrenaline and noradrenaline. These drug-like amines are usually either psychoactive or vasoactive. The psychoactive amines act on the neurotransmitters in the central nervous system while the vasoactive amines act directly or indirectly on our blood vessels. Examples of these biologically active amines include histamine, tyramine, serotonin, tryptamine, dopamine, and phenylethylamine. These substances are present in vegetables and fruit in fairly small amounts. They predominate in fermented food products including beer, wine, yeast extracts, fish such as tuna, meat extracts, beef liver, chicken liver, sausages, soy sauce, sauerkraut, and cheeses, as well as some vegetables like bananas and avocados.

The substance tyramine, which is derived from the amino acid tyrosine, is the most vasoactive substance. It constricts blood vessels and leads to a rise in blood pressure when large amounts are ingested. Tyramine is found in large amounts in various cheeses, yeast extracts, pickled herring, meat extracts and sausages. It acts pharmacologically by releasing noradrenaline from tissue stores, and this in turn causes an increase in the blood pressure. It is well known that patients who are taking antidepressant drugs, particularly the monamine oxidase inhibitors and similar drugs that decrease the breakdown of catecholamines, are not allowed to eat foods containing tyramine and other vasoactive amines which are found in yeasts, such as cheeses, pickled herrings, sausages and wines. The monamine oxidase inhibitors are antidepressant drugs which increase the tissue stores or noradrenaline, and thus potentiate the action of substances such as tyramine that might be found in these foods.

Many of these fermented food substances including wines, sausages, and cheeses are able to induce migraine attacks in susceptible people. It has also been shown in a controlled study in patients with migraine that 125mg of tyramine could produce headaches in 80 of 100 subjects, whereas lactose tablets produced headaches in only 6 out of 66 controls.

Other active amines that have been implicated in the production of migraine headaches include serotonin, phenylethylamine, and histamine. Phenylethylamine, like tyramine, causes an increase in blood pressure by liberating noradrenaline from tissue stores. Phenylethylamine has a potency of only 1/200 to 1/500th that of adrenaline, whereas tyramine has a potency of 1/20 to 1/50th the ability of adrenaline to increase

Table 9.1   Histamine and tyramine content of selected samples of food

Food product	Histamine (micrograms per gram)	Tyramine (micrograms per gram)
Beer and ale	not available	1.8–11.2
Cheeses		
Cheddar	0–1,300	0–1,500
Camembert	0–480	20–2,000
Emmenthaler	na	225–1,000
Brie	0	0–260
Blue or Roquefort	0–2,300	27–1,100
Cottage	0	0
Edam	0	300–320
Gruyère	na	516
Gouda	0–850	20–670
Mozzarella	0	0–410
Boursault	0	110–1,116
Provolone	10–525	38–150
Swiss	0	0–1,800
Stilton blue	0	460–2,170
Wines	0–22	0–25
Yeast extracts	210–2,830	0–2,256
Fish		
Tuna	2,040–5,000	na
Salted dried	na	0–470
Pickled herring	na	3,000
Meat		
Extracts	na	95–304
Beef liver	na	274
Chicken liver	na	100
Sausage	0.74–410	0–1,237
Soy sauce	na	1.76
Sauerkraut	7–200	20–95

Table 9.2   Biologically active amines in plant foods

Plant food	Tyramine	Serotonin	Tryptamine	Dopamine	Noradrenaline
Apple	—	—	0	—	—
Avocado	23	10	0	4–5	0
Banana peel	65	50–150	0	700	122
Banana pulp	7	28	0	8	2
Egg plant	—	0	0	—	—
Grape	0	0	0	0	0
Grapefruit juice	0	—	—	—	—
Orange	10	0	0.1	0	+
Passion fruit	—	1–4	—	—	—
Pawpaw	—	1–2	—	—	—
Pineapple juice	0.36	25–35	—	—	—
Plantain	—	45	—	—	—
Potato	1	0	0	0	0.1–0.2
Blue plum	—	0	5	—	—
Red plum	6	10	0–2	0	+
Red blue plum	—	8	2	—	—
Raspberry	13–93	—	—	—	—
Spinach	1	0	0	0	0
Tomato	4	12	4	0	0

blood pressure. The tyramine contents of various foods including cheeses, meat extracts and plant foods are shown in Table 9.1. High concentrations of tyramine (1–2mg/g) are present in cheeses and pickled fish but little tyramine is present in fruit and vegetables (Table 9.2). This might explain the numerous literature reports of hypertensive crises when foods have been eaten which include chocolate, yeast extract, liver (beef and chicken), broad beans and pickled herring. It appears that tyramine is always the major offender in precipitating these hypertensive crises. In man, 20–80mg of tyramine injected intravenously or subcutaneously will cause a marked elevation of blood pressure and in individuals taking monamine oxidase inhibitors as little as 6mg orally can cause a rise in blood pressure. It appears unlikely that the tyramine in fruits and vegetables could precipitate hypertensive attacks unless large quantities are consumed.

Histamine is derived from the amino acid histadine in the body, and it can also be formed during the fermentation process in many fermented or aged foods. It is a powerful capillary dilator, and causes hypotensive effects that lead to a decrease in blood pressure. It has been implicated in several outbreaks of food poisoning, especially after people have eaten fresh tuna, which can contain 200–500mg/100g. Gouda cheese has also been implicated; it contains up to 100mg of histamine per 100g. The histamine content of cheeses in general varies from 0–2,600mg/g. Usually if people ingest less than 225mg of histamine, there is no adverse reaction. However, some people are particularly susceptible and these are people with allergies, asthma, or perhaps peptic ulcers; they seem to react adversely to much smaller quantities. Following an intravenous injection of 0.1mg of histamine phosphate a person will experience facial flushing, an increase in pulse rate, a fall in blood pressure and a rise in the cerebrospinal fluid pressure, all occurring within twenty seconds. The onset of a histamine headache occurs one minute after injection. The symptoms of scombroid poisoning are similar to the physiological effects induced by histamine injection and these include nausea, vomiting, facial flushing, intense headache, stomach pains, burning sensation in the throat, dysphasia, thirst, swelling of the lips and urticaria. Although tyramine is the major precipitator of hypertensive attacks in patients taking antidepressant therapy, it has been found that the presence of histamine along with tyramine in yeast extracts or other foods such as fermented cheeses may alter the nature of the hypertensive attack. Monamine oxidase inhibitors facilitate the absorption of both tyramine and histamine from the intestine and potentiate their action. The presence of histamine could explain the occurrence of the persistent headache in hypertensive crises and the fall in blood pressure that is observed after its initial rise.

Chocolate is one food that has often been incriminated in hypertensive crises and it is suggested that vanillin, a catechol derivative, is the major precipitant. Chocolate is also known to contain substantial amounts of phenylethylamine. It has been shown that a two ounce bar of chocolate contains at least 3mg of phenylethylamine, but no tyramine. In this instance, phenylethylamine may be the dietary precipitant. Chocolate has also been implicated as a dietary cause of migraine headaches. When phenylethylamine (3mg) was given to individuals who suffered from migraine headaches precipitated by chocolate, 18 out of 36 individuals reported a headache. Only 6 out of 36 reported a headache after they were given a lactose placebo.

Tryptamine is another biologically active amine reported to be present in tomatoes, plums and other fruits and vegetables as well as cheeses. The levels of tryptamine reported in cheese vary from zero up to 1,100 micrograms/gram, generally lower than levels reported for histamine or tyramine. Although tryptamine has a pharmacological action similar to tyramine, there are no reports of tryptamine intoxication or of hypertensive crises.

Carbohydrate craving appears to be regulated by one of the chemical messengers in our brain called serotonin. This substance is manufactured from the dietary amino acid tryptophan and has been implicated as a possible cause of migraine headache, although there is no direct evidence. Serotonin is also present in fairly large amounts in bananas and other fruits and vegetables. While natural salicylates certainly appear to be a major factor in increasing hyperactivity in children eating high salicylate fruits and vegetables, it is possible that the large quantity of serotonin in bananas (see Table 9.2) may also play a role in learning difficulties in many children. It is also true that

Figure 9.1

Broccoli causes warfarin resistance
It is well recognised that increased vitamin K availability can antagonise the hypothrombinaemic effects of warfarin. This type of warfarin resistance is most frequently recognised in patients taking oral nutritional supplements containing vitamin K. However, as Sanford Kempin points out in a recent letter to the Editor of the *New England Journal of Medicine*, a high intake of a rich dietary source of vitamin K can cause similar problems. Green, leafy vegetables are the major dietary source of vitamin K, with vegetables such as turnip greens (650mcg/100g) and broccoli (200mcg/100g) having particularly high levels of the vitamin. In the two cases described by Kempin, a broccoli intake in excess of 230g/day was sufficient to produce warfarin resistance. In both cases, when broccoli was removed from the diet, prothrombin times were again prolonged to within therapeutic range by warfarin treatment.
(New England Journal of Medicine 308, 1229, 1983)

citrus fruits (which contain salicylates) contain active amines such as octopamine and synephrine.

Some individuals report intolerance to ripe or stored tomatoes but not to green ones. Later investigations have identified the active component of ripe tomatoes as a glycoprotein produced in the tomato skin by non-enzymatic browning reactions during ripening or storage. The component is resistant to heat and to trypsin and chymotrypsin, the two digestive enzymes found in the pancreas, so there is a high probability of its reaching the circulation after digestion. Of course, tomatoes, along with potatoes, eggplants, capsicum and all the other nightshades are also a family of foods that contain the active alkaloids solanidine and solanin, which have been implicated in arthritis.

In fact there are many naturally occurring plant toxins apart from the biologically active amines and some of these are listed in Table 9.3. In general, plant toxins are nature's 'pesticides'. Most people are probably ingesting several grams of these toxins each day, and levels of these natural insecticides and fungicides are specifically increased or decreased by plant breeders. There may be health costs associated with such human-control and manipulation of plant strains, just as there are for pesticides manufactured by man. Many plant toxins may cause indirect problems for humans after food animals consume plants containing these toxins. Cows and goats foraging on lupine (a legume which contains anagyrine) produce offspring with severe teratogenic abnormalities. Significant amounts of these teratogens may be transferred to the milk, so that human babies drinking the milk of such animals may be affected. Such a problem has already been reported in a rural Californian family, a baby boy, a litter of puppies and a number of goat kids. The problem was initially thought to be caused by the spraying of 2,4 D. Human exposure to fish, poultry, eggs and milk from animals fed on cottonseed may also give rise to potential problems. Toxic cyclopropenoid fatty acids (such as sterculic and malvalic acids) present in cottonseed become carcinogens in trout, cause atherosclerosis in rabbits and are mitogenic in rats. According to Dr. Bruce Ames, Chairman of the Department of Biochemistry at the University of California:

Table 9.3   Naturally occurring toxins in fruit and vegetables

Food	Toxin	Effect
Carrots	Carotatoxin Myristicin	Fairly potent nerve poison; hallucinogen (also in parsley)
Potatoes Tomatoes	Solanine chaconine (glycoalkaloids)	Cholinesterase inhibitor; interferes with transmission of nerve impulses; possible teratogens
Parsley Parsnip Celery	Psoralens	Produces photosensitivity, resulting in severe sunburning or tanning; psoralens also potential carcinogens and mutagens
Radishes Watercress Broccoli	Glucobrassicin Progoitrin Neoglucobrassicin Sinigrin Gluconoapin	Goitrogens, causing goitre
Avocado Bananas	Serotonin Dopamine Tyramine	Increase blood pressure; vasoconstrictors
Apples	Phlorizin	Glucosuria (glucose in the urine)
Oranges	Tangeretin (flavone) in peel, juice Tyramine Synephrine Citral	Embryotoxic
Rhubarb	Anthraquinines	Mutagenic effects
Herbs and herbal teas	Pyrrolizidine alkaloids	Carcinogenic, mutagenic, teratogenic
Broad beans (fava beans)	Vicine Convicine	Haemolytic anaemia in sensitive individuals (usually those of Mediterranean descent who have glucose-6-phosphate dehydrogenase deficiency)
Mustard seeds (mustard seed oil), horse radish	Allyl isothyiocyanate	Possible carcinogen and can cause chromosomal aberrations in animal cells
Alfalfa sprouts	Canavanine	Lupus erythematosus-like syndrome

For further information, see *Nutrition Today* 12, 6, November–December, 1977

The human diet contains a great variety of natural mutagens and carcinogens, as well as many natural antimutagens and anticarcinogens. Many of these mutagens and carcinogens may act through the generation of oxygen radicals. Oxygen radicals may also play a major role as endogenous initiators of degenerative processes, such as DNA damage and mutation (and promotion), that may be related to cancer, heart disease, and aging. Dietary intake of natural antioxidants could be an important aspect of the body's defense mechanism against these agents. Many antioxidants are being identified as anticarcinogens. Characterizing and optimizing such defense systems may be an important part of a strategy of minimizing cancer and other age-related diseases.

Another biologically active amine found in foods, particularly beverages, is caffeine. Caffeine is a methylxanthine, a potent

Figure 9.2

Danger of carrageenan in foods and slimming recipes

In a recent letter to the *Lancet*, R. Marcus and J. Watt from Chatterbridge Hospital, Cheshire, and Royal Liverpool Hospital, Liverpool, reiterated their warning about the long-term dangers of continued use of carrageenan and carrageenan-like products (Danish agar) in food, especially in slimming diets.

Referring to their earlier report on the harmful effects of carrageenan, based on observations in laboratory animals fed both degraded and undegraded (native) carrageenans as well as extracts of dried red seaweed from health food stores, they highlight the following results. Ulcerative disease of the colon was observed in rabbits and guineapigs fed 0.5–1% aqueous solutions of native carrageenan extracts from three different seaweed species. Undegraded carrageenan produced ulceration after two or three months, whilst degraded carrageenan produced the same effect within two to three weeks. Hyperplastic changes in the mucosa were frequently associated with the ulceration.

Whilst it has been claimed that carrageenan is neither digested nor absorbed, Marcus and Watt conclude that the bulk of evidence suggests the contrary, i.e. that carrageenan is absorbed in the gastrointestinal tract, and that high molecular weight carrageenans are degraded during their passage through the gastrointestinal tract and also as a result of food processing at acid pH and high temperatures. Only small amounts of degraded carrageenan (one part in 1000 in drinking fluid) are needed to produce ulcerative disease of the colon and hyperplastic polypoidal lesions in animals. The authors suggest that the toxic effects and tumour-enhancing properties of undegraded carrageenans observed in animals must be considered relevant to the use of carrageenan in foods. Despite interpretations to the contrary, these authors feel that the available data indicate the long term dangers in the use of carrageenan and carrageenan-like products in food.

(Letter, *Lancet* 8215, 11, 338 1981)

pharmacological agent. It is formed in many species of plant including coffee beans, tea leaves and cola nuts, and hence is found in most currently socially acceptable beverages, such as tea and coffee. It is also found in chocolates. It is the most popular and widely used stimulant drug in the world, and depending on the length of infusion, a cup of tea contains 50–80mg of caffeine and a cup of coffee 40–150mg. Lesser amounts are present in cola drinks. The pharmacologically active dose of caffeine is around 200mg, hence it is quite possible to produce clinical effects by taking large amounts of either coffee or tea and in susceptible individuals by only moderate amounts of these drinks. Caffeine is addictive and has widespread pharmacological actions which include the stimulation of the central nervous system and the heart and increased output of gastric acid and urine. It also has been found to dilate lung airways and is a bronchodilator. Some asthmatics have reduced their asthma attacks by taking many cups of coffee, as caffeine mimics the action of the asthma drug theophylline.

Caffeine toxicity can produce a clinical picture similar to a chronic anxiety state associated with tremor, palpitations, and rapid breathing. It can induce a state of palpitations due to extra heart beats called extrasystoles, or bouts of rapid heart beating called paroxysmal tachycardia. As a stimulant it can cause insomnia. Caffeine is also a vasoactive amine that may give rise to headaches. It is a potent inducer of migraine. If caffeine is withdrawn from migrainous subjects, the sudden withdrawal may lead to reactions such as severe headaches, irritability and lassitude. Large doses of both coffee and tea can produce nausea and vomiting in susceptible individuals. One of the earliest reports of caffeine-related side-effects was described in 1685. We now call this 'restless legs'. The principal sensations are an unpleasant creeping sensation in the lower legs between the knee and the ankle. This may have something to do with an induced vitamin B1 deficiency, and perhaps a buildup of lactic acid. The discomfort appears only at rest and usually in the evening or at night, and is associated with an irresistible need to move the limbs to obtain relief, hence the term, implying restless or jittery legs. The symptoms disappear after the caffeine has been removed from the diet. Because of the real risk of withdrawal reactions, caffeine should never be discontinued

166

Figure 9.3

The effect of caffeine on anxiety, plasma cortisol and MHPG levels in normal and panic disorder patients

A retrospective study of caffeine consumption by patients with panic disorder and normal subjects revealed that anxiety, alertness and insomnia were increased after consumption of 1 cup of coffee in the panic patients but not controls. Anxiety states in these patients were proportional to the amount of caffeine consumed, and for this reason 67% had ceased to consume coffee.

As anxiety has also been associated with noradrenergic function, a metabolite of noradrenaline; 3 methoxy-4-hydroxy-phenylethyleneglycol (MHPG), was monitored in response to a double-blind placebo-controlled caffeine challenge, as was cortisol (an indicator of hypothalmicpituitary-adrenal function) which is also associated with anxiety and lactate-induced and phobic panic. MHPG did not change with increasing caffeine consumption, although other studies have found that caffeine affects noradrenergic function. Cortisol levels however, in normal and panic patients increased with dose (480mg and 720mg) as did anxiety. Two normal patients experienced panic attacks after the 720mg dose accompanied by a 5 × increase in plasma cortisol. The pathogenesis of anxiety states could possibly be further elucidated by the use of caffeine challenges.

High doses of caffeine appear to induce anxiety states in normal and panic patients and is recommended that patients experiencing primary anxiety should minimise caffeine intake.

(Uhde, T.W., Boulenger J.P., Jimerson D.C., *et al.*, 'Caffeine and Behaviour: Relation to Psychopathology and Underlying Mechanisms. Caffeine: Relationship to Human Anxiety, Plasma MHPG and Cortisol'. *Psychopharmacology Bulletin* 20 3, 426–30 1984)

---

abruptly. Improvement of symptoms following withdrawal of coffee or tea does not necessarily prove that caffeine is the agent responsible because there are many other substances present in coffee.

One of the most recent effects to have appeared in the medical literature involves the emergence of anxiety neuroses and panic attacks in susceptible people following ingestion of large amounts of caffeine, either in the form of coffee or tea. These anxiety states and panic reactions arise after a large dose of caffeine increases the release of adrenaline, causing an increased metabolism of sugar and the formation of lactate. As lactate levels rise, so also does the anxiety and the panic attacks. Many patients with anxiety neurosis have been shown to have panic

Figure 9.4

> ### Caffeine poisoning elevates catecholamine levels
>
> N. Benowitz and other researchers (San Francisco General Hospital Medical Center), have described the metabolic changes which occurred in a patient who allegedly consumed 24g caffeine in a suicide attempt. The dose was far above that which was formerly thought to be lethal (10g).
>
> A peak serum caffeine level of 200mg/l was associated with massively elevated adrenaline and noradrenaline levels, as well as toxic levels of theophylline. The patient's severe hyperadrenergic syndrome included symptoms of haematemesis, tachycardia, hyperventillation, hyperglycaemia and ketonuria. Treatment with fluids and potassium gained a good response over 72 hours. The authors have suggested that β-blockers and perhaps α-blockers might be used in cases of severe caffeine poisoning, to counter the elevated catecholamine levels and adrenergic response.
>
> They have also recommended that the possibility of caffeine poisoning should be considered, as well as diabetes and salicylate poisoning, when patients appear with hyperventilation, metabolic acidosis, hyperglycaemia and peculiar behaviour patterns.
>
> (*JAMA*, 248, 1097–8 1982)

attacks after being infused with a solution of lactate. Other ways in which patients might inadvertently increase their lactate levels besides taking caffeine include the ingestion of alcohol and the sugars, fructose and sucrose. Lactate can also be increased by prolonged and strenuous exercise, especially anaerobic exercise which does not cause huffing and puffing.

While the great majority of people appear to be unaffected by the ingestion of reasonable amounts of food additives, including colouring agents and preservatives, naturally occurring biological amines, and other chemical substances present in foods, there appears to be a certain proportion of the population that is exquisitely sensitive to very small amounts of food additives. This has been shown by the Eggers group, Loblay and McGovern. Even very small (1mg or 1 microgram) quantities of substances such as dopamine may elicit hyperactive behaviour problems, while other chemicals might cause urticaria, gastrointestinal problems or increased heart rate in susceptible individuals. Many of these untoward effects may arise because the metabolism of the substances is inhibited or perhaps the metabolic enzymes necessary for their removal are genetically deficient or malfunctional. Whatever the reason for these adverse reactions, it is as important to consider chemicals that exist naturally in food as well as those food additives listed on the packets of processed foods, so that the consumer has a thorough understanding of the total number of reactive chemicals that are in the food, not just chemical additives and contaminants.

10

How do chemicals damage our body?

While I was working in the Chemistry Department at Macquarie University in Sydney, I produced a series of novel organic molecules which had potential application in the treatment of bronchial asthma; they were all related to adrenaline. By chemically modifying their aromatic part I could get much greater affinity of the potential drug for bronchial smooth muscle than cardiac muscle, hence minimising cardiac side-effects. Similarly, by chemically modifying the amine-containing side chain that hung off the end of these aromatic molecules I could change their overall activity. In this way medicinal chemists can increase the activity of a drug and also program the drug so that it selects one particular type of tissue.

By reacting many different types of chemical side chains with the basic molecular structure I was able to synthesise over two hundred different analogues (chemically related compounds). Most of them were related to adrenaline or one of the most common bronchodilator drugs called ventalin. In order to test them I took pieces of tracheal tissue or vas deferens from guinea pigs or isolated pieces of muscle from the guinea pig heart, placing them in a special solution together with the drug. By observing each compound's action on these isolated animal organs I was able to find out which particular new organic compounds were active on specific tissues and organs. These studies are called *in vitro*, the research being performed on isolated animal tissues rather than live animals. The one thing that struck me over and over again both with this *in vitro* work and also later with live animals (*in vivo*) was the fact that nearly every one of the two hundred compounds had some form of activity on one or more of the different types of tissue tested.

For many of these compounds the activity was only weak. Nevertheless the fact that such a vast array of structurally different compounds could elicit such a wide variety of pharmacological actions never ceased to amaze me.

The basic aromatic structure that I was working with, i.e. the benzene ring also called a phenyl group, is also the building block for thousands of different types of chemicals now used in our foods. For example, the preservative, benzoic acid, is an aromatic ring compound to which has been added a carboxylic acid. From benzoic acid we can get butylated hydroxyanisole (BHA) and butylated hydroxytoluene (BHT), both of these being preservatives. If we add a hydroxyl group to the aromatic benzene ring structure we get into the area of antiseptics. If we add a carboxylic acid and a hydroxyl group into the benzene ring we end up with salicylic acid, from which we derive the analgesic, aspirin and its analogue, methyl salicylate, which is commonly used in cough medicine, as well as the wide variety of salicylates that occur in fruits and vegetables to which some children are hypersensitive. If we go a little further and add another chemical group to the salicylic acid molecule we end up with drugs such as ventalin and an endless variety of related compounds such as those that I synthesised in the laboratory (see Figure 10.1). Most of these have some action on the many tissues of the body, especially the cardiovascular system and the lungs.

In a similar manner we can make organic compounds containing multiple aromatic ring structures containing phenyl groups and halogens such as chlorines or bromines to synthesise food additives which include erythrocine and tartrazine, many of the organochlorine herbicides, DDT, 2,4,5 T and others. By starting with a smaller molecule such as methane we can make chloroform and carbon tetrachloride, or we can oxidise it to make formaldehyde. By increasing the molecular chain length we can create ethanol (alcohol), propanol, butanol and eventually end up with the petrocarbon products to which many people are sensitive. These include drugs, dyes, explosives,

Figure 10.1   Structural similarity in aromatic compounds with diverse actions and uses

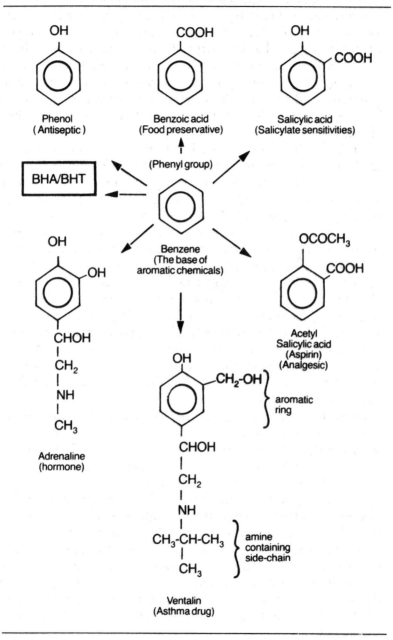

insecticides, plastics, detergents and synthetic fibres.

My first-hand experience in the laboratory as a medicinal chemist taught me that most of the compounds with which I was working affected some part of the body in a dose-dependent way, either pharmacologically or in a toxic manner. It was not surprising to me when I read in the literature reports of carcinogenicity, mutogenicity, teratogenicity, behavioural problems and chemical hypersensitivity reactions etc., which have now been linked to many of the above synthetic chemicals.

Many of these accumulate in the fatty tissues of our body, tend to destroy the liver or kidney and attack vital organs. If it wasn't for the complex detoxifying systems in our body we would quickly succumb to the foreign invasion of these agents which permeate our food and water supply. Because humans had been exposed long before the Industrial Revolution to many similar toxic chemicals that occur naturally in our food and environment, our bodies have developed a natural defence to help detoxify most toxins and foreign chemicals. Bodies are already used to accepting, chemically inactivating, and eliminating many chemical structures, but perhaps not some of the more recent novel compounds whose new chemical structures have never before been presented to our gene pool. We can handle synthetic chemicals in very small amounts but not when these start rising to such an extent that our inbuilt detoxifying mechanisms are overwhelmed.

Parallel with these changes we have also undergone a minor revolution in food production and processing which has significantly reduced the intake of food bound antioxidant nutrients which are intrinsically involved with detoxifying many of these chemicals. We are constantly engaging in enjoyable dietary practices (e.g. increased consumption of coffee, alcohol and sucrose) which place an undue load on the liver and the microsomal enzymes responsible for detoxifying.

So why is it that some individuals appear to be unaffected by environmental chemicals while others demonstrate extreme sensitivities ranging from behavioural disturbances right down the line to cancer? To answer this question let us examine some of the mechanisms that in general protect our body from chemicals.

Most people know that iron rusts when placed outside in the rain. Because of this we paint the iron with chrome or use galvanised iron. Fats similarly oxidise (or become rancid) if left for a considerable period of time in the air because oxygen attacks the unstable parts of the fat molecule, the polyunsaturated part. These same reactions also take place inside our body without some form of protection. In the oxygen-rich aqueous regions of our body we can oxidise minerals, and in our cell membranes the fatty substances, called lipids, become rancid unless both the minerals and the cell membranes are protected by specific enzymes and dietary nutrients called antioxidants. Both of these groups of protective substances make up the antioxidant defence system of our body which protects us from the equivalent of rusting or rancidity reactions within our body. The protective antioxidant enzymes involved in this system have names such as glutathione peroxidase, glutathione reductase, catalase, superoxide dismutase, and the protective dietary nutrients that act as antioxidants include vitamin A, vitamin E, vitamin C, beta-carotene and the minerals selenium, zinc, copper and manganese.

When single electrons are passed from one chemical species to another a so-called 'free radical' is formed. These are very destructive reactive species which can cause damaging oxidation in many of the areas of our body. These free radical mediated oxidative reactions are induced particularly by chemicals, herbicides, pesticides, solvents, drugs, radiation, foods, gases (such as sulphur dioxide and nitrogen dioxide) and heavy metals (e.g. mercury and lead). Such chemicals can also be converted to their free radical equivalents, which are very toxic and unstable, by the drug metabolising enzymes in our liver, kidney, lung and skin, and would eventually cause chemical hypersensitivity reactions, were it not for a strong antioxidant defence system in our body. The activated free radical forms of chemicals cause damage to tissue, inflammation and stimulation of the immune system, perhaps by the chemicals combining with proteins to form antibodies. All of these manifestations may accompany chemical hypersensitivity reactions in the body and other types of food allergy. These reactive free radicals with so-called 'unpaired electrons' also accelerate the production of dangerous superoxide anions. These are highly reactive oxygen

Table 10.1 **Our antioxidant defence system against chemicals (herbicides, pesticides, gases, drugs, toxic minerals), radiation, aerobic metabolism and autooxidation**

Protective enzymes	Protective antioxidants	
Glutathione peroxidase (requires selenium to activate)	Vitamin E Beta Carotene	Lipid solubles occur in cell membranes and in mitochondria
Glutathione reductase Glutathione transferase Superoxide dismutase (requires zinc, copper and manganese) Catalase	Ascorbic acid Uric acid	Water-soluble, occurs in blood and ascorbate in the CSF (cerebrospinal fluid)
	Ceruloplasmin (contains copper)	Accounts for 70% of antioxidant properties of blood serum together with transferin (which contains iron)

Vitamin E acts together with glutathione peroxidase in cell membranes to block lipid peroxidation which ultimately destroys a cell and contributes to the ageing of tissue. Ascorbic acid protects our blood, CSF, lung air spaces and other body fluids and acts synergistically at the membrane surface with vitamin E to produce an especially powerful antioxidant combination. Glutathione enhances ascorbic acid's antioxidant activity and they act together to protect vitamin E and beta carotene which in turn act to protect glutathione peroxidase which in turn acts to protect membrane lipids.

species formed by transferring single electrons from some activated chemical species to molecular oxygen in the body. Free radicals are also formed quite normally in the mitochondria, the cells' power houses, during cellular respiration, but are immediately disposed of.

So we can have activated free radical chemical species that have gained entry into the body (perhaps activated pesticides or food additives), and that are able to donate their electrons to oxygen to form a highly destructive form of oxygen called a superoxide anion. How can we protect the body from the toxic effects of superoxide anions? Firstly there are certain enzymes that are there to protect us against this activated oxygen species, called superoxide dismutase, glutathione peroxidase and catalase. The superoxide dismutase converts the superoxide anion to hydrogen peroxide by reacting two superoxide molecules with each other in a process which is called dismutation (see Figure 10.2).

Figure 10.2 Generation of free radicals and superoxide from chemicals

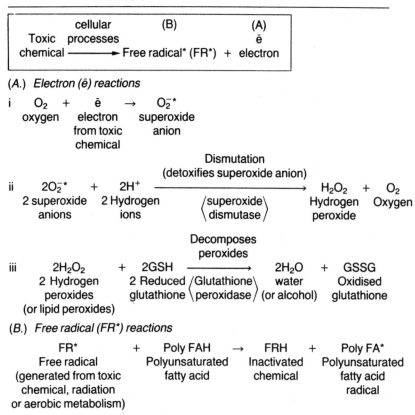

Free radicals are generated by toxic chemicals, aerobic metabolism, exposure to radiation or by autooxidation (not involving enzymes). These free radicals remove a hydrogen atom from a polyunsaturated fatty acid and form a fatty acid radical. This can initiate lipid peroxidation in cell membranes which can lead to their destruction if uncontrolled. Single electrons (ē) react with molecular oxygen to form the highly reactive superoxide anion radicals which can be inactivated by the enzyme, superoxide dismutase, to form hydrogen peroxide. This in turn is inactivated by glutathione peroxidase to form water. Otherwise hydrogen peroxide can form an even more reactive hydroxyl radical, and this activity is also dependent upon body supplies of selenium. Glutathione peroxidase activity rises quickly following an increase in selenium bioavailability. This is because selenium is an intrinsic part of the active site of glutathione peroxidase. So hydrogen peroxide (or other related organic peroxides) is reduced (the reversal of oxidation) by glutathione peroxidase to water. Glutathione peroxidase is not soluble in fatty environments but appears to be functionally associated with cellular membranes.

Superoxide dismutase is present in the mitochondria and also in the cytoplasm of the cell outside it. In the mitochondria the superoxide dismutase contains the mineral manganese, necessary to activate the enzyme. In the cytosol, the superoxide dismutase contains two subunits, each containing a copper and a zinc atom. So for the overall activity of superoxide dismutase we need copper, zinc and manganese. The hydrogen peroxide that is generated from the superoxide anion is, like all peroxides generated in our body, moderately toxic, and is further metabolised by either catalase or glutathione peroxidase. The catalase is fairly unimportant in human cells but the glutathione peroxidase is an enzyme that has the ability to inactivate peroxides, including a wide variety of lipid hydroperoxides, which are formed in the cell membranes. Glutathione peroxidase activity also becomes markedly elevated in response to an increased oxidative stress, such as the sudden intake of excessive amounts of toxic chemicals.

Many antioxidant nutrients are able to quench free radicals or active oxygen species. These include ascorbate (vitamin C), beta-carotene, cysteine, methionine, histadine, vitamin A and vitamin E. Uric acid and ceruloplasmin are two other antioxidant molecules which circulate in the blood. The circulating high-sulphur-containing amino acids such as methionine and cysteine, and ascorbic acid in the blood stream protect us from oxidation reactions in the aqueous areas of our body while beta-carotene, vitamin A and vitamin E (which are found in the lipids) protect us from membrane damage by lipid soluble-free radicals.

To give examples of free radical reactions, bromobenzene, as a free radical, can cause lung damage by binding to the lung tissue. Polycyclic aromatic hydrocarbons such as benzo-(a)-pyrene (found in barbecued meat), naphthalene and furan containing drugs are also activated, and their metabolites (chemically modified forms) are capable of donating the required electron, often changing the friendly molecular oxygen into the potentially toxic superoxide anion. In the lung, paraquat and nitro furantoin can also initiate free radical damage.

In order to modify the toxicity of these reactive oxidants, glutathione peroxidase needs a substrate (or food) for it to operate effectively. The name of this substrate is glutathione.

Elevated levels of these toxic substances will eventually cause a decrease in reduced glutathione, as it becomes oxidised or used up. For this reason it is necessary to have a good body supply of the three amino acids which are used to synthesise more gluta-thione. These are glutamic acid, cysteine, and glycine. All are important dietary components, when it comes to handling in-creased oxidative stress. The limiting amino acid is usually cysteine.

Glutathione peroxidase, glutathione transferase, catalase and superoxide dismutase are the main antioxidant enzymes in the lung. As these enzymes are all found inside the cell, ascorbic acid is left to play a very important role outside the cell. In fact, ascorbic acid may be the most critical component in the lung's defence against inhaled pollutants and metabolically active toxins. Damage to lung tissue by environmental chemicals is usually mediated by the free radical oxidising properties of the chemicals inhaled or taken in through the diet, or by free radical forms that are generated metabolically from them. These acti-vated small molecular weight-free radical chemicals can react with proteins to form hapten-protein complexes (the hapten being the chemical part of the complex). The hapten-protein complex then reacts with special cells such as mast cells or an antibody-forming cell to form specific antibodies, which on subsequent exposure of the hapten are released to fight or in-activate it. The antibody that is formed binds to the outside of the mast cells and basophils in such a way that when the hapten antigens next arrive, they combine with them to form what are called antigen-antibody complexes and at the same time imme-diately discharge the contents of these mast cells, which contain various allergy mediators including histamine, serotonin and leukotrines, initiating bronchoconstriction and perhaps even an asthma attack. (Intal acts by combining with and stabilising these mast cell membranes, preventing the release of the allergy mediators.) Because this immunological mechanism is at once activated, subsequent exposures only have to be very small to trigger it off, and this is why many patients with chemical sensitivities appear to react to such small amounts. They no longer react pharmacologically, in a dose-dependent way, or in an oxidative and destructive way; instead, the mere presence of a minute amount acts like a trigger which is recognised by the

Figure 10.3

Benzo(a)pyrene from barbecues
Charcoal grilling or open flame cooking of meats such as beef, chicken and pork causes them to become impregnated with a pro-carcinogen called benzo(a)pyrene in concentrations greater than 3μg/kg (Established safe limit 1μg/kg).   *(Journal of Agricultural and Food Chemistry* 31: 867 1983)

Cancer promoters and inhibitors
Natural unrefined whole food diets have a protective effect against cancer induced by carcinogen exposure, though some natural foods contain promoters and cocarcinogens and may be found in high concentration in animal protein and fat. Protective nutrients include ascorbic acid, vitamin E and selenium.   *(Nutrition and Cancer* 5: 107–19 1983)

immunological system and a whole cascade of immunological events follows, giving rise to various signs and symptoms which are recognised as being associated with chemical sensitivity reactions. The lung is usually equipped with plenty of antioxidant defences and when it senses an increased chemical oxidant attack it will increase the activity of a number of its antioxidant enzymes, such as glutathione reductase and glutathione peroxidase which decompose peroxides, and superoxide dismutase which detoxifies the superoxide anion. Glutathione levels rise and there is an increased activity in the selenium-dependent glutathione peroxidase and the superoxide dismutases.

We can add to this defence system, levels of free radical quenchers such as vitamin E and vitamin C, and many of the trace elements which are necessary for the production of these essential antioxidant enzymes. Usually this strong antioxidant system prevents many of the adverse reactions induced by these chemicals from occurring. When there are high levels of antioxidants there is no problem and 'tolerance' is usually developed. In other words, your body gets used to the familiar enemy and if enough nutrient antioxidants are present it can effectively fight the normal daily exposure of the specific chemical(s). However, if there is a depletion of the nutrient antioxidants, and a slow decrease in the activity of many of the antioxidant enzymes, then the tolerance that has developed is overwhelmed, and eventually the whole system breaks down. This explanation should also help us to see why many people have found that after a massive exposure to one particular type of chemical they can become intolerant to many other chemicals, even when exposed to them in very small doses. That is, the drain of antioxidant nutrients arising from one chemical leaves body defences weak and unable to cope with others. It also helps us to understand why middle-aged people suddenly become sensitive to chemicals. What happens is that their tolerance is breaking down as the ageing process progresses, and the antioxidant defence system in their body is slowly collapsing. Whether chemical hypersensitivity is caused by a direct inflammatory type of response to chemical oxidants or by an immune mediated response to a variety of chemical species, it is obvious that an affected person should strive for maximum activity of the antioxidant defence system.

Also particularly susceptible to oxidative damage are the endothelial cells that line arteries. This damage can be caused by heavy metal ions (mercury, lead, cadmium etc.), by activated chemical species, and also by lipid peroxides which can gain entry to the circulation from rancid dietary fats or from damaged tissues. As a consequence, pathological changes can occur in the membrane itself, causing cell death in the arterial walls; this can lead to atherosclerosis. It is presently thought that the particular target organ or tissues that are likely to be attacked by a reactive chemical species is in many respects the result of genetically determined biochemical weaknesses to which these individuals are predisposed. There are two basic mechanisms that are thought to account for membrane damage due to toxic chemicals. The first is lipid peroxidation and the second, direct bonding of a chemical or its reactive metabolite to the membrane itself. Most tissue damage is thought to be free radical mediated.

Metabolites of foreign chemicals can also be extremely toxic, either due to their high reactivity as radicals, usually having a tendency to form chemical bonds with biomolecules or to their ability to convert molecular oxygen into free radicals. In the latter case superoxide and other oxygen anions then mediate oxidative stress to the tissues. When laboratory mice are

exposed to sublethal doses of ozone, they become tolerant very
quickly to it. They also develop a cross-tolerance to other oxidant gases including nitrogen dioxide and phosgene. Tolerance
is manifested biochemically as increased activity in protective
antioxidant enzymes such as glutathione peroxidase (GP), and
also its support enzymes, glutathione reductase (GR) and glu-
cose-6-phosphate dehydrogenase (G6PD). These three become
elevated in rat lung tissue. Whether they are reduced or not in
response to the oxidant gas load will depend a lot on nutritional
factors, e.g. whether there is enough selenium in the diet, it
being a co-factor of glutathione peroxidase. A further question
is whether there are enough sulphur-containing amino acids
such as cysteine and methionine in the diet, since these are
components of glutathione. Even though tolerance can be
maintained for a short period, over a long period of time
chronic degenerative effects are observed in mice, including
chronic lung degeneration, premature ageing and in one particular cancer-susceptible strain, lung tumour acceleration.
Hence, the oxidative stress, if it continues, leads to deterioration of the systemic antioxidant capacities of an organism and
finally a state of exhaustion. When this is reached, it is often
associated with inflammatory symptoms and depressed immune function. It is the final stage of what Hans Selye has called
General Adaptation Syndrome. The first stage represents acute
exposure to a stress, the second is one of adaptation to it, and
the third and final stage is one of exhaustion and degeneration
when tolerance breaks down.

Animal studies have also shown that our bodies have a mar-
vellous ability to increase the activity of antioxidant enzymes
such as glutathione peroxidase in those tissues where there is
greatest oxidative stress and not in others. For example, when
rats are fed a corn oil diet that is deficient in vitamin E, the
activities of GP, GR and G6PD are increased in several adipose
tissues and in the muscle in proportion to the abnormal elevation of liver peroxides in them, but the activities of enzymes do
not increase in liver, lung, kidney and other organs where liver
peroxides are not found to accumulate.

In two disorders of the blood called sickle cell anaemia and
thallasaemia, there is much peroxidative damage. In both, the
superoxide ion is produced in much greater quantities then

normal. Peroxidative changes occur in the polyunsaturated fatty acids in the red cell membranes and eventually red cells are destroyed. Red cell glutathione peroxidase levels are elevated both in sickle cell anaemia and in thallasaemia, and the red cell glutathione peroxidase activity increases adaptively as there is an elevation in oxidative stress.

Studies of normal subjects exposed occupationally to chemicals have found that they, compared with controls who had not been exposed, had a much lower selenium status. Smokers had a much lower level of selenium and GP activity in erythrocytes. GP activity is generally lower in many systemic diseases. Red cell GP activity and selenium levels are lower in patients with Down's Syndrome, skin disorders and head and neck cancers. Schizophrenics have been shown to have elevated lipid peroxides and lower red cell glutathione peroxidase levels. Elevated lipid peroxides have also been found in patients with skin burn injury and also diabetes and stroke.

Dr. Stephen Levine, an American researcher exploring chemical hypersensitivity reactions, has suggested that the development of adaptive tolerance to oxidative stress in one organ can deplete or reduce antioxidant reserves elsewhere in the body. He says 'many powerful pharmaceutical agents will contribute to oxidative stress upon their metabolic activation to react with radical derivatives by mixed function oxidase and other enzyme systems. Individual genetic predispositions will likely dictate our unique resilience to oxidative stress and determine which tissues and organ systems are particularly susceptible.'

When the body is subject to an acute oxidant stress it calls for an immediate reinforcement from other reserves in the body which may already be low. This is why some crisis situation will happen frequently in an adult, and even though he may get through a fairly rough episode, following this, the body may be seen to deteriorate. This is because the organ reserves of antioxidant nutrients and specific enzyme activities will be depleted, and systemic reserves exhausted.

Levine has cast new light on Hans Selye's General Adaptation Syndrome. He now sees four stages of progression of chronic diseases related to the onset of chemical exposure. In stage one the individual is in good health and protected against oxidant stresses. Then suddenly he is exposed to the toxic chemicals that are proliferating around us. The body acts resiliently. Then stage two is entered, adaptation to oxidative stress. In this, the individual has to compensate for various life stresses. He might be subject to oxidative stresses from situations such as breathing polluted air, living with a leaking gas stove or heating system, or being exposed to chemicals at work or to pesticides in the garden. This extra chemical exposure draws more on the antioxidant defences required to handle life stresses and eventually to some degree they compromise overall resistance to disease and sense of wellbeing. Stage three incorporates losing the struggle, and the emergence of clinical disease symptomatology. At this stage signs of chronic and acute illness appear: inflammatory damage occurs to the more genetically susceptible organs and reactive oxidising chemical species cause the liberation of allergy mediators and other mediators of inflammation such as kinins, histamines and serotonin. All these are liberated as a consequence of uncontrolled chemically induced membrane (peroxidative) damage. Finally the stage of exhaustion sets in, where antioxidant defences are severely damaged by oxidant stresses and perhaps nutritional deficiency.

Over the last twenty years, of the many millions of chemicals reported in scientific literature, it is estimated that 50,000 are presently in current use: pesticides, fertilisers, herbicides, food additives, household chemicals, industrial chemicals and drugs. All must undergo detoxification in our body and they do so in many cells of our organism with the aid of drug and chemical-metabolising enzymes. The organ that appears to be most important for metabolic detoxification is the liver. Some of the major drug-metabolising enzymes are found in special areas of the liver cells called hepatocytes known as the endoplasmic reticulum. They are also called the microsomal enzyme system, often referred to as cytochrome P450-dependent-mixed function-oxidase, and, more simply, mixed function oxidases (MFO). This MFO system catalyses the initial deactivating metabolic changes to lipid soluble foreign chemicals that enter our body so that they can be subsequently conjugated (chemically bonded) with small organic molecules, making them more water soluble for excretion through the bile, the faeces or the urine. These chemicals are water-solubilised by combining with substances such as glutathione, glucuronic acid, taurine or glycine, or by the transfer of sulphate, methyl or acetyl groups to the hydroxylated foreign chemical metabolite. When environmental chemicals, either as gases, water or foods, enter the system, they 'induce' (activate or turn on) the mixed function oxidase system, the MFO system. Chemicals that are known to activate the detoxification system are dioxins, DDT, chlorinated hydrocarbon insecticides, urea herbicides, polycyclic aromatic hydrocarbons, polychlorinated biphenyls (PCBs), aromatic isothiocyanates, and other naturally occurring food toxins.

The MFO system is also swiftly brought into action by naturally occurring chemicals in many of our dietary vegetables such as broccoli, cabbage, cauliflower and other green leafy vegetables. When these vegetables have been fed to experimental animals such as rats, they have been protected against hepatic toxicities induced by concomitant exposure to potent chemical carcinogens such as polybrominated biphenyls and even aflotoxin. Usually the MFO system takes these chemicals and rapidly activates them, generating reactive-free radical metabolites. These are short lived because the free radical species are rapidly scavenged and inactivated. Hence these reactive intermediates do not usually tend to accumulate. However, sometimes the system becomes overloaded and reactive chemicals can accumulate. Because of this, activated chemicals that

Figure 10.4

Organochlorine research

Organochlorines are bioactivated by liver enzymes rather than being detoxified and excreted. The resulting epoxides and peroxides cause membrane damage and lead to formation of free radicals which can in turn interact with DNA to act as mutagens.

Nakayama, T. *et al. Agric. Biol. Chem.* 48: 571–2 (1984); Reynolds, E.D. *et al.* In *Free Radicals in Biology*, Vol. IV, W.A. Pryor, ed. NY: Academic Press (1980)

Organochlorines restrict the movement of minerals across cell membranes and inhibit cellular respiration. Lindane specifically inhibits the energy generating centre of cells.

Nelson B.D. *Biochem. Pharmacol.* 24: 14385–390 (1975); Gopolaswamy, U.V. *et al. Bull. Environ. Contam. Toxicol.* 35: 106–13 (1984)

have gone through this system and have not been properly deactivated can cause abnormal metabolic problems: altered protein synthesis, chronic inflammatory reactions and auto-immune reactions. They can also chemically react with DNA molecules causing changes in our genetic material that can result in mutagenic and carcinogenic effects.

Many chemicals are known to actually *inhibit* the MFO system. These include organophosphorous insecticides, carbon tetrachloride, carbon monoxide, ozone and heavy metals. A low-protein diet can be particularly damaging because the protein supplies the amino acids, glycine, taurine, glutamine, and cysteine, which are involved in deactivating the activated chemicals. Most chemicals are easily detoxified and rapidly eliminated from the system. However, if the liver is exposed to large levels of a chemical metabolite, it can become increasingly more toxic because it depletes the liver of essential protective nutrients, particularly reduced glutathione. Many chemicals can end up generating superoxide or hydrogen peroxide, because the activated chemical species has a free electron which it can donate to oxygen. Examples of compounds that do this (called redoxcycling) are compounds containing benzene rings, such as phenols and aromatic nitrate compounds, pesticides, such as Paraquat, and antitumour antibiotics such as adriomycin. Some of these activated metabolites can actually bind directly to detoxifying enzymes such as P450 cytochrome and can cause the whole detoxification chain to be disrupted. This again leads to abnormal generation of superoxide in the membranes and eventually a disruption of the internal structure of the cell. This is one of the major mechanisms of chemical toxicity in the liver. Examples of substances which can inactivate the P450 enzyme by binding directly to it include carbon tetrachloride, halothane, amphetamine, sulphur-containing pesticides such as the fumigant, carbon disulphide, and the cholinesterase inhibiting insecticide, parathion.

Carbon tetrachloride is one chemical that is found every-where in the environment and its highly reactive metabolite, CCl_3 is highly toxic to the liver. Carbon tetrachloride can cause lipid peroxidation but this can be protected against by antioxidants such as vitamin E. Much of the chloride added to our drinking water can also become toxic because it reacts in

Figure 10.5

Treatment of carbon tetrachloride poisoning
Acetylcysteine treatment has been used to minimise hepatorenal damage arising from carbon tetrachloride poisoning. Acetylcysteine supplies an additional source of the sulphur containing amino acid cysteine which is converted into the enzyme glutathione peroxidase which in turn helps to remove toxic peroxides formed by the carbon tetrachloride.
If acetylcysteine is not available, animal studies have provided some evidence that vitamin E and selenium may act synergistically to protect against carbon tetrachloride hepatotoxicity. This alternative should be considered in cases of human poisoning.
Yurdakok M., Yurdakok K., Caglar M. Institute of Child Heath, Hacettepe University, Ankara, Turkey, Letter, *Lancet* 1: 1336 (1985)

ground water with organic material to form chlorinated hydrocarbons such as chloroform and dichlorobromomethane which can also be found in drinking water. The hypochlorite ion is another toxic species that can be formed by combination of chlorine with water; it can further combine with phenolic compounds present to form phenyl chlorides which are structurally similar to the insecticide, DDT, and chlordane.

Excessive intake of alcohol can also adversely affect the liver causing peroxidative damage. This can be protected against by having ready availability of some of the antioxidant compounds such as selenium, but the induction of liver MFO by alcohol can also potentiate the hepatotoxic effects of other chemicals such as vinyl chloride, and the analgesic paracetamol, and also phenobarbital, which is a barbiturate. One of the major adverse effects of chronic alcohol consumption is the fact that it reduces the level of many of the antioxidants in the body. There is a definite depletion of water-soluble and fat-soluble antioxidant nutrients in the liver. There are lowered levels of magnesium, calcium, copper, zinc, manganese and selenium, and chronic alcohol intake has also been found to cause malabsorption of thiamine, folic acid, vitamin B12, many of the amino acids, and the fat-soluble vitamins A, D, E and K. Therapeutic administration of these key nutrients, in particular vitamin E and ascorbate, together with the sulphur amino acids, cysteine and methionine, can protect against the deleterious effects of both

186

Figure 10.6

Dietary selenium protects against paraquat toxicity

The LD_{50} of the herbicide Paraquat (PQ) in chicks deficient in vitamin E and selenium, was increased threefold by 0.1ppm dietary selenium. Supplementation with vitamin E (100 IU/kg diet) did not significantly affect the LD_{50} of PQ. Increasing the fat content from 4% to 20% of the diet did not affect the toxicity of PQ; however, exposure to an oxygen enriched atmosphere slightly reduced the protective effect of dietary selenium.

Maximum protection against PQ toxicity in chickens was achieved by dietary sodium selenite higher than 0.04ppm; however, levels above 0.08ppm were needed to show a detectable increase in plasma glutathione peroxidase.

Effects of vitamin E and selenium on the toxicity of paraquat *Nutrition Reviews* 42(7): 260–2 (1984)

---

acute or chronic alcohol intake. Alcoholics are also advised to avoid caffeine, cigarettes, sugar and other substances which tend to increase free radical generation.

Many of the plant foods that we eat on a daily basis contain toxic chemicals in fairly large amounts. These chemicals are produced by the plants as natural pesticides or insecticides for defence against bacteria, fungus, insects and other animal predators. The compounds are often chemically related to the common industrially produced pesticides, and other environmental pollutants. Examples are the pyrolisidines that are found in comfrey, saffrol which is found in black pepper, sassafras which is a potent carcinogen in mice, aflatoxins which are produced from the aspergillus mould, and many other compounds such as phenols, quinone and catechols, all of which are capable of generating free radical and activated species of oxygens in our body.

Most of the common prescription drugs that we get from the local pharmacist are also detoxified through the liver. These include paracetamol, adriamycin amitriptyline, chlorpromazine, dilantin, hydrazines, imiprimine, methotrexate, phenobarbitol and tetracycline to name a few. Paracetamol, for example, is usually quickly combined with glutathione and excreted. However, small amounts can be converted by the MFO system to a very toxic metabolite, called NABI (N-actyl-

Figure 10.7

BHA and potassium bromate link with cancer
The subject of food additives is a controversial one at the best of times, but recently Japan has decided to restrict the use of the food antioxidant, butyl hydroxy anisole (BHA) and also potassium bromate which is used in the treatment of flour. The restriction of both chemicals is near enough to a complete ban, following toxicological studies revealing that 29–35 per cent of rats developed oesophageal cancers after eating a diet containing 2 per cent BHA. Potassium bromate was associated with renal cancers. Other European countries are studying these results closely and may follow suit. Some countries have already banned potassium bromate as a food additive. *(European Chemical News 7 June 23 1982)*

parabenzoquinone imine) and if the liver glutathione levels are low or the person has been fasting, this metabolite tends to react chemically with proteins in liver cells, often killing the cell. Acute and chronic paracetamol toxicity problems have been successfully treated using antioxidants, glutathione, N-acetylcysteine, cysteine, methionine and vitamin E. When glutathione levels are reduced in the liver by fasting, the toxicity of many drugs such as paracetamol are increased. The toxicity of paracetamol in fasted animals, for example, increases eightfold; that for another chemical, bromobenzene, increased twenty-five fold, correlating with a reduction in the levels of reduced glutathione. The mutagenic and carcinogenic properties of adriamycin have been shown to be protected against by α-tocopherol (vitamin E).

In 1976 I was working in the New York State Department of Health, Albany on the east coast of the United States. At that time there was an uproar about the PCBs (chlorinated aromatic hydrocarbon compounds) that were being dumped into the Hudson River and consequently were being picked up by fish and contaminating the food chain. PCBs were being used as major constituents of insulating oils for electrical utility transformers. Unfortunately, the PCBs are very poorly metabolised. They tend to accumulate in living tissues, especially in body fat, from which they are released when fat is broken down during weight reduction or fasting, and also during milk production in the pregnant woman. A United States government survey carried out in 1980 revealed that 30 per cent of mothers' breast milk had levels of PCBs above 0.05ppm; in Michigan, half the nursing mothers surveyed had milk levels of PCBs higher than 0.06ppm. Neurological and developmental impairment in children up to nine years of age has been associated with PCB contamination of breast milk. PCBs are also potent immune suppressors and carcinogens.

As we have already discussed, another substance which is highly toxic, widespread throughout the environment, and not able to be metabolised to any great extent in humans, is dioxin. This is a contaminant in many PCBs and also the herbicide 2,4,5T, (Agent Orange). Exposure to dioxin has resulted in liver damage, skin cancers, psychological derangement and impaired functioning of the immune system, both in test animals and in humans suffering from inadvertent exposure.

In 1983 Lassiter and co-workers examined the tissues of 200 chemically hypersensitive patients for 16 different chlorinated hydrocarbon pesticides. They found that most of the patients, or the average patient, had about 3 to 4 different pesticides each with blood levels usually in parts per billion. The levels in other tissues could have been higher. It was demonstrated that 1ppb of dieldrin in the blood is equivalent to 158 parts in adipose tissue, 26.3 parts in liver, 4.9 parts in brain white matter and 3.3 parts in brain grey matter. This really is showing that the blood levels of organic compounds can significantly under-represent their levels in other tissues. DDT was also found in 62 per cent of patients. It is a potent inducer of MFO. Incidentally, none of the patients had any occupations concerned with the manufacture of these chlorinated hydrocarbon pesticides.

Lassiter found that the serum of ill patients contained many other chemicals, which included benzene, toluene, stylene, chloroform and tetrachloroethylene, which were detected in greater than 1ppb, in twenty-four patients tested. Trimethylbenzene, bromoform, trichloroethane and trichloroethylene were also detected in more than half the patients tested.

Chlorinated hydrocarbon pesticides levels were also found to be high in Germany, in both adults and children, comparable with levels found in the United States and in Hawaii, where the contamination has filtered through to the ocean and is now sufficiently concentrated to cause severe skin outbreaks in

Figure 10.8

Phenoxy herbicides and cancer

A *Lancet* report from D. Coggon and E. Acheson (MRC Environmental Epidemioiogy Unit, University of Southampton at Southampton General Hospital, Southampton) and a follow up editorial in the same issue, have evaluated all the available evidence from Sweden, the United States, Finland and New Zealand linking phenoxy herbicides, chlorophenols and their contaminants with the incidence of soft tissue sarcomas and lymphomas in workers who manufacture or use these compounds in agriculture. They have concluded that while the results of the few studies so far made are conflicting, there seems to be sufficient and urgent cause for more extensive and controlled research, especially since these herbicides continue to be of invaluable use in forestry and agriculture, and even less is known about the toxic potential of available substitutes.

The phenoxy acid herbicides include 2,4,5-T and 2,4-D which were constitutents of the Agent Orange defoliant used in Vietnam, as well as MCPA, 2,4-DP, and MCPP. Among the suspect chlorophenols, used as wood preservatives and herbicides, are 2,4,5-trichlorophenol, pentachlorophenol, 2,4,6-trichlorophenol, and 2,3,4,6-tetrachlorophenol. The most toxic of the dioxins which contaminate all of these compounds is TCDD (2,3,7,8-tetrachlorodibenzoparadioxin). TCDD is found in 2,4,5-T and 2,4,5-trichlorophenol, and its maximum allowed limit in Britain is 0.01mg/kg. Before 1965, 2,4,5-T contained as much as 30mg/kg.

In 1977, seven patients from a Swedish oncology clinic, with soft tissue sarcomas, gave case histories which suggested exposure to unspecified doses of again mostly unspecified phenoxy acid herbicides at some time over a 10–20 year period. As a result two case-control studies were begun to compare exposed patients with tumours to unexposed control patients.

In the first study, in heavily forested northern Sweden where the suspect chemicals were frequently used, the relative risk estimated for exposure to 2,4,5-T and 2,4-D combined, and to chlorophenols was 5.7. It was impossible to estimate a risk factor from exposure to single chemicals, since insufficient evidence was available.

In the second study, in southern Sweden, where the herbicides are used for agriculture rather than in forestry, a similar study established a risk ratio for exposure to be 5.1. There was no significant relationship found between degree or length of exposure and the risk ratio.

While four further studies (two in Sweden, one in Finland and one in New Zealand, admittedly on small numbers of patients and without long-term follow-up, have failed to establish similar results, there have been published data on the high incidence (given the rarity of these cancers in the population as a whole) of soft tissue sarcomas in American workers involved in the manufacturing of phenoxy acids and

Figure 10.8   (Cont'd)

chlorophenols. Heavy exposure to TCDD seems to produce a form of dermatitis termed chloracne in these workers. Since the number of workers in this industry is small, the incidence of soft tissue sarcomas seemed quite high. Three further studies of similar workers in Germany and Czechoslovakia have detected no deaths from soft tissue sarcomas.

Problems encountered in collecting and assessing information included insufficient information on the nature and length of exposure, unreliable recall of events by relatives and friends, and imprecise histological data on the nature of these rare tumours. Nevertheless, with all present evidence considered, the authors have concluded that it seems possible that the occurrence of soft tissue sarcomas may be related to exposure to phenoxy herbicides and chlorophenols, or to the contaminant TCDD (and there is mounting evidence that this dioxin is carcinogenic in animals). They suggest that levels of TCDD be kept as low as in Britain and that further data should be collected and assessed as soon as possible, using measurement techniques newly available for detecting levels of phenoxy herbicides and related compounds in the blood and urine of exposed workers.

Lancet 1, 1057–9 (1982) and Editorial, *Lancet* 1, 1051–2 (1982)

swimmers. Fortunately, many of the micronutrients that we consume daily play a very important role in detoxifying these chemicals and safeguarding our body from extensive damage. When rats are fed carbon tetrachloride or ethanol, if they are also fed vitamins A, E, ubiquinone, vitamin C, vitamin B12 and choline, these nutrients protect against the enhanced lipid peroxidation and other cellular pathology normally produced. It is also interesting to note that carbon tetrachloride causes a decrease in the liver levels of vitamins B1, B2, B3, vitamins A, E, and ascorbate. The fact that many of these chemicals can induce the MFO system is in one way an advantage, because low background levels of the chemicals lead to a more effective detoxification when increased quantities of chemicals are present. But at the same time it can also lead to overload from toxic accumulation, leading to depletion of local supplies of antioxidants such as ascorbic acid, glutathione and alpha tocopherol (vitamin E). Without these nutrients to protect many of the cellular enzymes, there would be wholesale destruction of the entire chemical defence network. Often a combination of many different types of chemicals in small amounts can overwhelm the capacity of the MFO system. This puts an enormous drain on the antioxidant defences. In this way the whole detoxifying system of the liver is highly sensitive to dietary deficiencies of antioxidant nutrients. If the MFO function is impaired, for example, by a deficiency of vitamin E, there is an increased toxicity of many drugs and chemicals. When rats are deprived of vitamin E they are unable to detoxify (hydroxylate) pheno-barbital. However, when resupplemented with vitamin E, they are again able to hydroxylate the drug, and there is also a con-comitant lowering of the drug's toxicity. Similarly, a deficiency of ascorbate (vitamin C) in experimental animals leads to a de-crease in their ability to detoxify many of the chemicals that become substrates (food) for the MFO.

We have already spoken about the important role of reduced glutathione as a helper for glutathione peroxidase but in the MFO system it is particularly important because it is one of the major conjugating agents leading to deactivation of chemical metabolites, which can be quickly excreted in either bile or urine. Prolonged fasting leads to a decrease in serum and tissue levels of glutathione. A combination of a low-protein diet or fasting will therefore increase the oxidative stress on many chemically hypersensitive patients and this is one of the reasons there are violent reactions (adverse symptoms) when chemical-ly hypersensitive patients (with an overload of chemicals) start to fast. Low-protein levels or fasting lead to lower levels of the amino acids, glycine, taurine and cysteine, so the production of glutathione would be decreased. Many of the conjugation reac-tions (detoxification) that take place in specialised liver cells (called parenchymal cells) would also be decreased.

Selenium has been shown to be one of the most important minerals for the liver's detoxifying ability with respect to elevated PCBs in rats. It works together with other antioxi-dants such as vitamin C and vitamin E to maintain a very active functional detoxification system.

In summing up, it can be seen that a sufficient supply of amino acids is critical for the person suffering from chemical hypersensitivity reactions. This means that we should make sure of a good daily supply of protein, otherwise we cannot make the glutathione which requires adequate levels of cysteine, glycine and glutamic acid. With sufficient glutathione at hand, ample conjugation can take place with reactive metabolites of chemicals to render them water soluble, so that they can be excreted in the urine. Vitamins C and E are also important in the detoxification process, for regulating the inducibility of the MFO system, and selenium because it is an integral part of the glutathione peroxidase enzyme.

11

Food allergy versus chemical sensitivity

**What are the differences between food protein
and peptide allergies and chemical hypersensitivity
or toxicity?**

Let's take chemicals first. The intake of these from herbicides,
food additives, drugs and other sources can cause direct damage
to tissues and be toxic to enzyme systems, or they can become
pharmacologically active like drugs or hormones to cause
changes in metabolic events, by acting at receptors on cell
membranes. All toxic chemicals are also changed by drug-
metabolising enzymes in the liver, kidneys, lung and skin, to
become free radical metabolites of the parent compounds.
These toxic metabolites can then attack the cell membrane
lipids, by causing peroxidation and the generation of free
radical fatty acids both in the outer and inner membranes of the
cell. The free radicals so generated can start up a chain reaction
unless they are quenched by the ready availability of fat-soluble
nutrients in the brain such as vitamins A, E, beta carotene and
the membrane-containing enzymes such as glutathione peroxidase. These reactive chemical species can also interact with key
amino acids, particularly those containing sulphur like cysteine,
methionine, histadine and tyrosine, thereby inactivating or
changing enzyme activity. They can also interact with the
structural and functional proteins containing these same amino
acids (reactions with immunoglobulins cause deficits in im-

193

mune function). They can interact by binding to nucleic acid bases which are the building-blocks of our genetic material, DNA and RNA. All of these changes consequently may lead to abnormal metabolic processes, incorrect protein synthesis, mutations, autoimmune antibodies, chronic inflammation and so on. Quite apart from this effect of the intake of foreign chemicals, free radical intermediates are continually being produced in the body and cause the formation of superoxide, hydrogen peroxide and hydroxyl radicals. They are also formed through processes of cellular respiration (that is, oxidative phosphorylation to produce ATP), intermediary metabolism via oxidase and dehydrogenase enzymes and phagocytosis by macrophages and neurophils, and, in addition, during the production of inflammatory mediators, prostacyclins, thromboxanes and prostaglandins from the precursor fatty acid, arachidonic acid. They are all examples of cellular metabolic mechanisms which generate free radicals in both health and disease.

Manifestations of chemical hypersensitivity usually indicate that the adaptive enzyme systems responsible for producing chemical tolerance in an individual are not operating or are malfunctional. It also may indicate that many of the antioxidant nutrients such as ascorbic acid, beta carotene, vitamin E and glutathione, are deficient, due to restricted dietary intake, or the inability of a person to regenerate the biologically active forms of these antioxidant nutrients. Hypersensitivity reactions to very small amounts of a chemical (often multiple chemicals) usually indicates that a small chemical called a hapten is mediating the hypersensitivity reaction.

The hapten combines with a protein to form a hapten-protein conjugate which is subsequently recognised as foreign by the immune system so that an antibody is produced against it. Subsequent exposure to the chemical hapten can produce immediate hypersensitivity reactions as the result of the antigen-antibody induced disruption of a mast cell or basophil, containing various chemicals such as histamine, leukotrienes and serotonin. These substances are involved in inflammation, swelling and pain, as well as many of the acute symptoms associated with such chemical hypersensitivity reactions. The other possibility is that a chemical might react with a protein in such a way that it changes the structure so that the body recognises it as foreign and the same type of immunological process as just described is undertaken where this protein suddenly becomes an antigen, and goes through the same immunological and biological process of antigen removal.

A good example of immune mediated chemical or drug sensitivity is the occupational asthmatic who has been exposed to toluene diisothiocyanate. In this particular case there is a latent period between the initial sensitising exposure to the chemical and the hypersensitivity reaction. During the initial exposure hapten-protein complexes are formed which stimulate the production of the hapten specific antibodies which subsequently bind to lung mast cells and basophils. The typical asthmatic response is elicited by re-exposure to the chemical. Acute respiratory hypersensitivity signs and symptoms ensue. This clinical response is not related to the pharmacological or oxidant properties of the drug or chemical and may be precipitated by exposure to very small quantities of the sensitising agent. So chemical hypersensitivity may be initiated either by direct exposure to strong toxic chemicals or by immune mediated mechanisms similar to those seen in chemical or drug pulmonary hypersensitivity reactions.

In the case of a food allergy we have a completely different mechanism. The offending food particle is usually a protein or a part thereof called a peptide. These fragments can arise from eggs, fish, chicken or indeed any protein food. They are absorbed unhindered through the wall of the gastrointestinal tract. In other words they escape digestion by our normal digestive process including the digestive enzymes in the wall of the small intestine, and gain entry into the body. In some cases the digestive process can actually generate these reactive substances in the gastrointestinal tract. As soon as these foreign molecules are recognised as such by the body they are called antigens and induce the formation of antibodies (immunoglobulins, usually IgE). When these IgE type antibodies are formed, they are able to combine with the antigen (the peptide or protein) and this combination reacts at the surface of a mast cell to stimulate its bursting open and the release of various allergy mediators, such as histamine. This type of reaction is called an immediate hypersensitivity reaction because the signs and symptoms attendant on it are usually immediate. But there can also be delayed allergic reactions involving other immuno-globulins which can take many days to manifest. Many migraine sufferers come under the delayed category; a particular reactive food consumed for breakfast one morning may not show up until two or three days later as a migraine headache.

So both food proteins/peptides and also the low molecular weight chemicals, haptens, can participate in immunological reactions which are termed food allergies or, in the case of haptens, chemical hypersensitivity. The great majority of adverse food reactions are related to small chemical molecules which are associated with foods, but are not proteins or peptides, and which can cause toxic reactions through the formation of reactive free radicals or by acting directly on tissues in the same manner as drugs.

12

How we can cope with food chemicals

We cannot just remove ourselves from our environment without disrupting our lifestyle. It is not always convenient to move house, place of employment or from one city to another. Besides, industrial chemicals and their byproducts now pollute all life on this earth; there is no escaping the intake of chemicals by skin, lungs or stomach. So what can we do about the situation? How can we cope if we feel that these substances are adversely affecting our health?

Firstly, it is necessary to reiterate that our bodies have been taking in pollutants and food toxins for thousands of years. As shown, most simple vegetables have naturally occurring toxins, such as solanidine in tomatoes, and such substances are capable of producing free radicals in our bodies which could attack our tissues were it not for our antioxidant chemical defence systems, especially in our liver and kidneys, inactivating toxins and other contaminants found in our food and water supply. Even some of the more novel chemical compounds synthesised in laboratories around the world which eventually end up in our bodies are still successfully handled by the various detoxifying units stationed throughout our bodies, though of course some synthetic chemicals are more toxic than others. Usually chemicals with carbon–chlorine or carbon–fluorine bonds in the molecule (such as carbon tetrachloride), or aromatic compounds containing chemical bonds (such as DDT) are much harder to process and are far more toxic, possibly because our gene pool

197

has never been exposed to these latter compounds and specific detoxifying mechanisms in our tissues have not been elaborated over the past thousands of years. In other words, our bodies feel that the 'toxins they know are better than the toxins they do not know'. *So firstly, we need to minimise our known exposure to such agents.* Minimise does not mean remove completely, which is an impossibility! Minimise means to actively avoid where possible by gaining more knowledge about the chemical environment in which we live, and then acting on this information by making careful selections of foods, household goods, etc., or else performing certain procedures which reduce the impact of the chemicals.

The following approaches should be considered when dealing with suspected food chemical sensitivity.

Herbicides and pesticides

Minimise the effect of herbicides and pesticides by choosing non-sprayed products if available. Choose food that is fresh and seasonally growing. Don't eat fruit or vegetables out of season and you immediately remove yourself from the impact of the agents used to delay ripening, prolong shelf life, preserve colour and texture, etc. Special fruit and vegetable washing solutions are on the market to help remove the spray residues and these may be helpful for some sensitive individuals. Peeling fruit and removing the outer layer of some vegetables also considerably reduces the total chemical residue burden of the food. Organochlorines on apples and cucumbers, for example, defy even rubbing and washing, so peeling is the only appropriate choice. Peeling pears removes the high salicylate areas and allows a salicylate-sensitive individual to eat an otherwise restricted food.

Food additives

Not all food additives are harmful. Something with a long chemical sounding name does not necessarily mean that it is a villain; many people tend to mistakenly equate the length of a name with its toxicity. The consumer must now be ready to recognise immediately which chemicals may be harmful simply by reading available consumer leaflets and becoming fully acquainted with the properties, uses and other relevant characteristics of the chemicals being consumed.

Carboxymethyl cellulose, which sounds like a sure carcinogen, is simply an inert component of fibre. Food acids such as citric acid and tartaric acid or their salts, sodium citrate and sodium tartrate, are harmless metabolic products produced by every cell of our bodies and found also in most fruits. They are completely harmless food additives and must be identified as such by the consumer and contrasted to known trouble-makers such as tartrazine and erythrocine, and also other substances which have continually turned up in clinical trials as suspect agents in chemically related disorders (i.e. MSG, benzoic acid, sodium metabisulphite, etc.). Look for the chemical food additive name and/or identifying code number on packets of food. Choose only foods with additives you know will cause you no adverse reactions. In the beginning it is wise to eliminate all foods containing food additives for at least three or four weeks.

Naturally occurring food chemicals

Some reactive agents such as natural goitrogens or alkaloids are found in many members of the same family of foods. Solanine, a glycoalkaloid, is found in many members of the nightshade family (tomatoes, potatoes, eggplant, capsicum). Goitrogenic substances are found in the celery and mustard families (carrots, cabbage, and broccoli). It is therefore wise to check with Food Family tables to see if there is a pattern of adverse reactions arising from members of the same family. If you are reacting to two or three members, it may give you a clue as to the nature of the reactive chemical. It may then be wise to avoid all members of that family for a definite period of time. It should also be remembered that not all food family-related reactions are due to chemicals. Some may be due to the protein components (notably gluten which occurs in foods containing wheat, rye, oats and barley); others may simply be a problem of fat intolerance if the foods are high in fat, or an allergic reaction to one of the proteins in cows milk, or an intolerance to milk sugar (lactose). This area has already been covered in my book *Food Intolerance — What it is and how to cope with it* (Harper & Row, 1984).

If you are trying to detect a chemical sensitivity, remove all alcoholic beverages, caffeinated drinks and foods containing xanthines (i.e. chemicals related to caffeine) such as coffee, tea, cola drinks, chocolate and cocoa and in many cases herbal teas and food spices which contain an abundance of naturally occurring plant drugs. Carefully consult the tables of foods containing salicylates or the biologically active amines, tyramine, dopamine, noradrenaline, phenylethylamine, serotonin and tryptamine. Avoid fermented foods or foods containing moulds or yeasts and always try to obtain fresh foods. Frequently naturally occurring food chemicals are formed as the food freshness is lost. This is particularly evident with fish and other seafoods.

Fasting for detoxification purposes

Fasting on pure water can cause a rapid release of chemically related toxins from body tissues due to their movement from tissue stores and lymphatic clearance into the blood stream. Fat tissue and major body organs store most fat-soluble chemicals, and bone is the major storage site for lead, and an important one for aluminium. A safer approach is to use a modified fast. After first checking with a nutritionally enlightened doctor, try four or five days on raw juices, raw salad vegetables, sprouts, vegetable soups and fruits such as pawpaw (papaya) and watermelon. The best juices to use are mixtures of carrot, beetroot, celery, cucumber and spinach with apple or pineapple as a base and with small quantities of parsley and radish.

After four days or more, depending on how you are feeling, sprinkle an equal mixture of sesame, sunflower and pumpkin seeds (roasted and ground) into your soups or onto your salads and introduce a little homemade yoghurt (preferably goat's yoghurt) each day for the next three or four days. You may then introduce eggs which contain the high sulphur amino acids, methionine and cysteine, and cold water fish which is high in the essential oil, eicosapentaenoic acid (EPA). If you introduce grains use *non*-sprayed brown rice. All legumes such as lentils, kidney beans, chick peas and other beans should be soaked overnight and the water changed three times during cooking. During the early stages of your modified fast you will be rapidly moving chemicals from the liver, skin and kidneys. This accelerated turnover increases your requirement for anti-oxidant nutrients, which should be taken as extra supplements during this time and continued later on. You should also start a light aerobic exercise program, or perhaps take up yoga or *tai chi* classes or use a mini-trampoline to help the movement of the lymphatic discharge into the blood stream. Lymphatic and liver drainage massage techniques and also intestinal massage may be necessary for some and should be carried out under the supervision of a qualified health professional who will also advise you on the use of substances such as kaolin, bentonite and activated charcoal or perhaps D-penicillamine, or chelation therapy in the case of heavy metal poisoning.

During the first week or two it is necessary to drink plenty of fluid to help remove conjugated chemicals through the kidneys. Before and after the actual juice fasting stage, regular bowel movements are essential. If this poses a serious problem it may be advisable to start the fast by taking Epsom salts ($Mg SO_4$). A high-fibre alternative is to take one or two tablespoons of raw linseeds before bed each night, washed down with plenty of warm water. This latter method is especially suitable because the linseeds are a food. They have no harsh laxative effect, but swell up in the gastrointestinal tract to give bulk; they are also highly fibrous and mucilaginous and contain important nutri-ents which include the Ω-3 fatty acid alpha-linolenic acid. Alternatively, some people find it most effective to take one small teaspoon of ascorbic acid each hour for several hours until the bowels become loose and then drop back on the dose to about a teaspoon every 4–5 hours until the end of the day. All these methods should be started only after checking with your local health professional and should be accompanied by plenty of pure drinking water.

After the first couple of weeks of mainly juices, vegetables and fruits, a more balanced diet should be entertained, but at least one day each week should be set aside as a 'juices only' day and the rest of the week should still rely heavily on fresh raw foods with similar macronutrient ratios to those suggested by Pritikin, i.e. about 80 per cent complex carbohydrates, 10 per cent protein and 10 per cent fat. Don't overeat. It is most important not to overload your digestive capacities. You can increase the effectiveness of your digestive enzymes by taking smaller mouthfuls, chewing well and getting up from the dinner table feeling just short of satisfied.

Adverse reactions may occur during the first week of the fast. These may include nausea, vomiting, diarrhoea, headaches, boils, eczema, dandruff, foul-smelling stools, joint and back pains, increased heart rate, shakiness, confused thinking, and extreme fatigue. Some of these symptoms are due to mobilisation of stored chemicals into the bloodstream, while others may be 'withdrawals' after removing the offending food or foods; these may be helped by taking a teaspoon of mixed alkali salts in a glass of water, followed by another full glass of water. This procedure should be carried out approximately a half to one hour after eating and the alkali mixture should consist of two parts sodium bicarbonate to one part potassium bicarbonate. Do not take this mixture more than twice in one day and take strictly as directed and not at the same time as ascorbic acid (which will react with the bicarbonate).

Protective diets for Russian workers

The Russians have always taken an active interest in nutrition and over the past thirty years have developed five different dietary rations for workers in toxic chemical occupational environments. Each of these provides about 1,400 Kcal and consists of 16–18 per cent protein, 26–33 per cent fat and 46–55 per cent carbohydrate; each is designed to decrease the harmful effects of chemical exposure (see Table 12.1). Dietary Ration No. 1 is designed for workers exposed to radioactive substances and x-rays and is the only one that includes fresh fruit. Rations Nos. 2 and 3 have fewer dairy products and are used to protect workers against exposure to cyanide compounds, nitric and sulphuric acids, chromium oxides, fluorides and lead. Ration No. 3 is specifically aimed at preventing lead

Table 12.1 **Recommended list of foods and quantities for Soviet workers in toxic chemical occupational environments**

Food (quantity in g)	Ration no. 1	2	3	4	5
Rye bread	100	100	100	100	100
Wheat bread	—	100	100	100	100
Wheat meal	10	15	4	15	3
Cookies	—	—	50	—	—
Zwieback	5	—	—	—	—
Grain, pasta	25	40	45	15	20
Beans	10	—	35	—	—
Green peas	—	10	—	—	—
Sugar	17	35	32	45	40
Meat	70	150	130	100	100
Fish	20	25	50	50	35
Liver	30	25	25	—	25
Eggs‡	3/4	1/4	—	1/4	1
Kefir§	200	200	—	200	200
Milk	70	—	—	—	—
Cottage cheese	40	—	—	110	35
Sour cream	10	—	—	20	10
Cheese	10	25	—	—	—
Animal fat	20	15	25	15	17
Vegetable oil	7	13	—	10	15
Potato	160	100	—	150	125
Cabbage	150	150	—	—	—
Carrots	90	—	25	25	100
Tomato purée	7	2	3	3	3
Fresh fruit	130	—	—	—	—
Cranberries	5	—	—	—	—
Tea	0.4	0.5	1.5	0.5	0.5

‡ Portion of egg
§ Slightly effervescent acidulous beverage from cow's milk
Source: Okorokova Yul, Yeremin Yul N., *Hygiene of Nutrition.* Meditsina, Moscow, 1981, as compiled by E. Sutphen, *American Journal of Clinical Nutrition* 42: 747, 1985

uptake and has very low calcium content. After ten days on this low calcium ration the worker is switched to Ration No. 2 or 4. Ration No. 4 is used where there is exposure to aromatic amines, nitrobenzenes, chlorinated hydrocarbons (organochlorines), arsenic compounds, phosphorus and tellurium, Ration No. 5 is used against organophosphorus pesticides, carbon disulphide, mercury compounds, magnesium and barium.

All of these dietary rations are aimed at influencing the absorption, tissue distribution, cell interactions, detoxification and elimination of environmental toxins. Supplemental vitamins are also used where appropriate. Vitamin A (2mg) and

204

Table 12.2   Examples of recommended vitamin(s) and amounts for Soviet workers subjected to different chemical exposures or working conditions

Chemical exposure/working conditions	Vitamin(s) administered
Fluorine, chlorine, cyanide, and alkali metals	Vitamin A (2mg) Ascorbic acid (100–150mg)
Arsenic, tellurium, tetraethyl lead, bromine hydrocarbons, carbon disulfide, thiophos, mercury, and manganese dioxide	Thiamine (4mg)
High temperatures (e.g. breadmaking industries) and nicotine dust (tobacco industries)	Vitamin A (2mg), thiamine (3mg), ascorbic acid (150mg) and nicotinic acid (20mg)
Noise	Ascorbic acid (quantity not specified)
Vibration	Ascorbic acid, thiamine, riboflavin, and nicotinic acid (quantities not specified)

Source: Sutphen, as Table 12.1.

ascorbic acid (100–150mg) are used against fluorine, chlorine and cyanide exposure and thiamine (vitamin B1, 4mg) against mercury, arsenic, tellurium, tetraethyl, lead, bromine hydro-carbons and carbon disulphide, for example (see Table 12.2).

Water purifiers

A good water purifier may also be money well spent if water contamination is a major problem. It should be able to carry out three entirely different functions. Firstly, it should be able to filter out solids — all particulate matter down to the smallest particle. Secondly, it should be able to remove the small amounts of organic solvents present in the water supply, including herbicides and industrial pollutants. Activated charcoal is often used for this purpose. Finally, the purifier should contain a special resin capable of removing minerals (cations) such as lead, mercury, aluminium and copper and non-minerals (anions) which include chlorine, fluorine, phosphates, sulphates and sulphites. Check with the manufacturer to ensure that these three criteria are fulfilled.

Antioxidant nutrition supplements

If the free radicals arising from chemicals or drugs are not inactivated by the body's detoxification mechanisms, they damage tissue. They set up a chain reaction (called lipid peroxidation) in the polyunsaturated fats in cell membranes. They inactivate important enzymes in our bodies and also combine with our genetic material which may lead to damaged and malfunctional metabolic processes.

To protect cells from the deleterious effects of lipid peroxidation, we need adequate levels of beta carotene, vitamin A, vitamin E, glutathione peroxidase and its activating trace mineral, selenium. This group of antioxidants protects cell membranes from chemical attack because they are fat soluble and are found in the cell membranes themselves.

The liver is possibly the most important organ for detoxifying drugs and chemicals. As previously mentioned, the key enzymes in it are the cytochrome P450 oxidases and mixed functioning oxidase enzymes. The cytochrome P450 enzymes take the chemical and make it more water soluble through a process called hydroxylation. The hydroxylated chemical ions then combine with glucuronic acid, glutathione, sulphate, glycine or taurine, or can be otherwise chemically modified by methylation or acetylation. This modified water-solubilised chemical is not only less toxic than the original molecule, but is quickly eliminated through the kidneys. The key to the successful modification of these chemicals depends upon dietary availability of substances such as taurine, glycine, glutathione or precursor molecules into which they can be converted in the body. The cytochrome P450 oxidases are located on specialised membranous structures (endoplasmic reticulation) inside liver cells and are regulated by levels of corticosteroids (e.g. cortisone) and vitamin E. Vitamin E deficient animals cannot initiate the cytochrome P450 dependent water-solubilisation process so necessary for elimination of chemical toxins. It appears that vitamin E protects the lipid containing membranous structures inside the cell whose integrity is required for cytochrome P450 oxidase activity.

Superoxide dismutase (SOD) is the enzyme responsible for destroying the dangerous superoxide radical that can be generated by exposure of the body to various chemicals. There are two different types of SOD in human tissues. The first has two identical subunits and is found in the cytoplasm of the cell. It contains one atom of zinc and one atom of copper per subunit. The other form is also found in mitochondria (the power houses) of each cell and contains the trace mineral, manganese. Zinc, copper and manganese are critical for the functioning of SOD, as they constitute the active site of the enzyme. Hence the importance of an adequate dietary supply of these minerals.

Glutathione peroxidase which forms the final and probably the most important defence barrier against membrane lipid peroxidation contains four atoms of selenium per mole (molecular weight expressed in grams) and uses up glutathione (composed of the amino acids, glutamic acid, cysteine and glycine), every time it has to dispose of hydrogen peroxide or lipid peroxides. Hence the importance of selenium and a plentiful supply of the glutathione precursor amino acids. Several heavy metals such as mercury and cadmium are known to lower glutathione peroxidase activity by interacting with selenium. Selenite, an inorganic salt of selenium, and vitamin E have been shown to reverse the toxic effects of mercury.

The importance of the trace elements zinc, copper, manganese and selenium for activating these enzymes which catalyse the destruction of free radicals, thus providing our primary defence mechanism, cannot be overemphasised. It also follows that deficiency of one or more of these minerals can seriously compromise our chemical defence system. The elaborate enzyme systems are inherently leaky, however, and allow reactive free radicals to escape. For this reason there is a powerful secondary defence screen of small antioxidant molecules patrolling our blood stream — vitamin E, ascorbic acid, beta-carotene, glutathione and ceruloplasmin. Ceruloplasmin accounts for approximately 70 per cent of the blood's antioxidant properties, with transferin, an iron-containing protein, also contributing. Ceruloplasmin is activated by copper. It inhibits lipid peroxidation and is a scavenger of free radicals. Another group of small proteins called metallothionines bind heavy metals such as cadmium, mercury and lead with high affinity. Metallothionine contains about 30 per cent of the amino acid, cysteine. Exposure to toxic heavy metals increases

Figure 12.1

Allergic reactions to contaminants in water

When an ubiquitous consumable like water is contaminated with allergens the effects are insidious and evade diagnosis. In persons concurrently allergic to a food or pollen, attempts at allergen desensitisation and food exclusion diets are foiled.

The initial reaction of the target organ to an allergen is stimulation, an energy consuming process. (During this period the patient is more sensitive to cold.) This is followed by a depressive phase. After chronic exposure to an allergen, affected cells lose their capacity to respond. This cessation in activity may be temporary or permanent. Elimination of the allergen from the environment results in a withdrawal syndrome with exacerbation of the symptoms. These general principles apply when the allergen is a water contaminant.

The target organs for water bound allergens are mostly the ones that come into contact with water: skin, eyes, nose, alimentary canal and the urinary system. But the musculo-skeletal and nervous systems (both central and peripheral) have also been involved. The symptoms seen in people allergic to water contaminants include the following: irritability, dizziness, insomnia, inability to concentrate, tiredness, skin inflammations, excessive thirst, bed wetting (in children), urinary urgency, dysuria, haematuria, vaginal, penile and anal irritation,diarrhoea, constipation, asthma, headache, greasy and itchy or dry scalp with falling hair, pain in neck, shoulders and calves of legs, bleeding gums and salivation or dry mouth with ulceration. Some of the apparently incompatible symptoms are produced at different phases of the allergic reaction. The behaviour of these people when dealing with water (e.g. baths) is also contradictory, some avoid water and some are addicted to it.

A group of 10 children in Ireland were diagnosed as being hypersensitive to tap water by the use of food sensitivity analysis, water sensitivity analysis and skin prick tests; and by observing the persistence of symptoms after two months on a food exclusion diet (the diet was supplemented with vitamins for the second month). The effects of antigen on taste and sensory fibres proved to be a sensitive and accurate test for diagnosis. At this point a complete water exclusion therapy was commenced.

Children experienced typical withdrawal symptoms during the first 4–14 days; during the second and third months a definite improvement was observed. The alimentary and urinary tracts showed the fastest improvement. Tissues from which the allergens only could be disposed of by metabolic processes improved more gradually. Upon rechallenge a deterioration in symptoms was observed within 30–60 minutes.

The author indicates neutralisation therapy to be the next step in treatment.

Wilson, C.W.M. Law Hospital, Carluke, Lanarkshire, Scotland, *Nutrition and Health* 2, 51–63 (1983) metallothionine levels in the kidney, liver and spleen. Both cysteine and zinc also stimulate the endogenous production of this important detoxifying protein.

Minerals compete with each other for uptake into the body and binding to various proteins and enzymes. For this reason, oral doses (or increased dietary levels) of specific antagonistic minerals can be used therapeutically to lower the body burden of toxic mineral contaminants. Zinc supplements taken orally are known to compete with copper, cadmium and iron, and have been used to reverse toxic manifestations of excess copper or cadmium body burdens. Zinc supplements have been used to decrease the high copper levels associated with Wilson's Disease. Blood aluminium levels have been successfully lowered with supplemental zinc, manganese and magnesium. Calcium supplements together with ascorbic acid have been effective in lowering an increased lead burden.

Throughout the scientific literature there are numerous studies supporting the use of the above vitamins, minerals, amino acids, peptides and other specific antioxidants for the treatment of problems arising from environmental chemical exposure. Ascorbic acid has been used for scavenging nitrosamines and carcinogenic compounds formed after exposure to benzo(a)pyrene. Acute and chronic acetoaminophen (drug) toxicities in humans have been treated with glutathione, N-acetylcysteine, L-methionine and vitamin E. Ethanol and carbon tetrachloride-induced pathology is prevented by administration of oral vitamins A, E, C, B12 and choline. Increased dietary methionine has protected against the toxic effects of methyl mercury hydroxide (a neuro toxicant) and atrazine (a herbicide). Daily supplementation of healthy elderly subjects with 400mg vitamin C, reduced lipid peroxide levels by 13 per cent in one year, and when vitamin E (200mg daily) was also added the lipid peroxide levels were reduced further, to about 25 per cent.

All the studies to date indicate that an increased oral intake of the major antioxidants and specific minerals not only offer protection against low background exposure to herbicides, pesticides, drugs, food additives, heavy metals and other sources of environmental exposure but also can be used in the treatment of adverse reactions arising from the exposure to such agents. These protective nutrients are shown in Table 12.3.

Table 12.3   Daily supplemental doses of some major nutrients required for optimising the protective antioxidant defence system

Minerals (elemental values)		Vitamins		Amino acids	
Zinc	20mg	Ascorbic acid	2g	Methionine	300mg
Copper	5mg	Vitamin E	250mg	Cysteine	300mg
Iron	15mg	Vitamin A	10,000i.u.		
Manganese	5mg	B-complex	20–50mg		
Selenium	200mcg		(approximate values		
Molybdenum	5mg		only and excluding		
			vitamins B12 [250mcg]		
			folate 250mcg, biotin		
			100mcg)		

Note: Supplemental β-carotene, taurine, N-acetycysteine, glutathione may also be beneficial in certain circumstances and after obtaining professional advice

While some food chemicals will always prove to be a problem for susceptible individuals, an increased awareness of the situation together with a thorough knowledge of the differences between one chemical and another, between the potentially harmful ones and those that are safe, gives us greater control over food selection by allowing us to avoid naturally occurring food toxins as well as specific food additives. Increasing concern over food and water contaminants has also resulted in the greater market availability of organically grown foods. When these are not available or their purchase proves impractical, there are still the special washing solutions for fruit and vegetables already mentioned, and a variety of different types of water purifiers to choose from. It must be pointed out, however, that one of the most basic ways of reinforcing our body's defences against food chemicals is often simply a matter of eating *only* fresh, highly nutritious, well-balanced foods which are high in complex carbohydrates, fibre and antioxidants with adequate protein and essential oils and low in animal fat. To this minimum requirement we can then add supplemental antioxidant nutrients which are known to play a very important role in our body's defences against chemicals in general.

Finally, the whole approach to food chemicals boils down to four considerations — knowledge, avoidance, neutralisation and detoxification — all, of course, within the limitations dictated by our inherited constitution.

References

Allen, D.H. 1985. Environmental factors in the provocation of asthma and hay fever. *Australian Family Physician* 14(3): 172–6.

Allen, D.H., Van Nunen, S., Loblay, R. *et al.* 1984. Adverse reactions to foods, Special Supplement. *The Medical Journal of Australia* S37–42.

Ames, B.N. 1983. Dietary carcinogens and anticarcinogens. *Science* 221: 1256–64.

Anderson, J.A. 1984. Non-immunologically mediated food sensitivity. *Nutrition Reviews* 42(3): 109–16.

Augustine, G.J., Jr., and Levitan, H. 1980. Neurotransmitter release from a Vertebrate neuromuscular synapse affected by a food dye. *Science* 207: 1489–90.

Batagol, R. 1984. Drugs and Breast feeding. *Australian Pharmacist* November: 18–22.

Bryce-Smith, D. 1980. Lead or Health. London: The Conservation Society Pollution Working Party.

Buist, R.A. 1984. *Food Intolerance: What it is and how to cope with it.* Harper & Row, Sydney.

Cant, A.J., Gibson, P., and Dancy, M. 1984. Food hypersensitivity made life threatening by ingestion of aspirin. *British Medical Journal* 288: 755–6.

Capaioannou, R., and Pfeiffer, C.C. 1983. Sulfite sensitivity — unrecognized threat: is molybdenum deficiency the cause? *J. Orthomol. Psychiatry* 13(2): 105–10.

Carson, R. 1982. *Silent spring.* Pelican Books.

Cawcutt, L., and Watson, C. 1984. *Pesticides: the new plague.* Collingwood, Victoria, Australia: Friends of the Earth.

Choice, Journal of the Australian Consumers' Association. December 1985. Antibioties and you.

Collins, J.A. 1984. Roadside lead in New Zealand and its significance for human and animal health. *New Zealand Journal of Science* 27(1): 93–7.

Commonwealth Department of Health, Canberra, Australia. 1985. Standard for maximum residue limits of pesticides, agricultural chemicals, feed additives, veterinary medicines and noxious substances in food. Ninety-eighth Session of the National Health and Medical Research Council, October 1984.

Connell, D.W. 1981. Water pollution — causes and effects in Australia and New Zealand. St Lucia, Queensland: University of Queensland Press. Australia.

Cope, I., Stevens, L., and Lancaster, P. *et al.* 1975. Smoking and pregnancy. *The Medical Journal of Australia* 2, 745–7.

Davies, D.P. 1976. Gray, O.P., Ellwood, P.C. *et al.* Cigarette smoking in pregnancy: Associations with material weight gain and fetal growth. *Lancet* 1: 385–7.

Delohery, J., Simmul, R., Castle, W.D. and Alan, D.H. 1984. The relationship of inhaled sulphur dioxide reactivity to ingested metabisulphite sensitivity in patients with asthma. *Am. Rev. Respir. Dis.* 130: 1027–32.

Denner, W.H.B. 1984. Colourings and preservatives in food. *Human Nutrition: Applied Nutrition* 38A: 435–49.

Dormandy, T.L. 1983. An approach to free radicals. *Lancet* 2, 1010–14.

Driscoll, W.S., and Horowitz, H.S. 1978. A discussion of optimal dosage for dietary fluoride supplement, a Report of the Council on Dental Therapeutics, American Dental Association. *J. Am. Dent. Assoc.* 96: 1050.

Egger, J., Carter, C.M., Graham, P.J., Gumley, D. and Soothill, J.F. 1985. Controlled trial of oligoantigenic treatment in the hyperkinetic syndrome. *Lancet* 1: 540–5.

En-Trophy. 1980. Modern agriculture: destroying the soil to people link? 1–16. *Institute Review* 3(2).

Feingold, B.F. 1975. Why your child is hyperactive. New York: Random House.

———, Behavioural disturbances linked to the ingestion of food additives. New dynamics of preventive medicine. 1977. In Medical progress through innovation, ed. Leon R. Pomeroy. Vol. 5. International Academy of Preventive Medicine.

Ferguson, A.C. 1984. Food allergy in progress in food and nutrition. *Science* 8: 96–7.

Florence, T.M. 1983. Cancer and ageing. The free radical connection. *Chemistry in Australia.* 50(6): 166–74.

Freundlich, M., Abitol, C., Zilleruelo, G. *et al.* 1985. Infant formula as a cause of aluminium toxicity in neonatal uraemia. *Lancet* 2: 527–9.

Garattini, S. 1979. Evaluation of the neurotoxic effects of glutamic acid. In *Nutrition and the Brain*, eds R.J. Wurtman and J.J. Wurtman, 79–124. New York: Raven Press.

Gibson, A. and Clancy, R. 1980. Management of chronic idiopathic urticaria by the identification and exclusion of dietary factors.

Clinical Allergy 10: 699–704.

Gilchrist, A. 1981. Foodborne disease and food safety. American Medical Association, PO Box 821 Monroe. WI. 53566.

Greene, G.R. 1976. Tetracycline in pregnancy. *New England Journal of Medicine* 295(9): 512–13.

Hall, R.H. 1984. *Food for Naught*. Sydney: Harper & Row.

Hall, R.L. 1977. Safe at the Plate. *Nutrition Today* 12(6): 6–31.

Hanson, M. 1983. Amalgam — hazards in your teeth. *J. Orthomol. Psychiatry* 12(3): 194–201.

Hanssen, M. 1984. *E for additives — the complete E number guide*. Wellingborough, Northamptonshire: Thornsons Publishers.

Holmes, A. 1984. Role of food additives. *Chemistry and Industry* 6 February: 104–7.

Huggins, H.A. 1982. Mercury: a factor in mental disease. *J. Orthomol. Psychiatry* 11(1): 3–16.

Hunter, B.T. 1980. *Additives Book*. New Canaan, Connecticut: Keats.

Juhlin, L. 1981. Recurrent urticaria: clinical investigation of 330 patients. *British Journal of Dermatology* 104: 369–81.

King, D.S. 1984. Psychological and behavioural effects of food and chemical exposure in sensitive individuals. *Nutrition and Health* 3(3): 138.

Lafferman, J.A., and Silbergeld, E.K. 1979. Erythrosine B inhibits dopamine transport. In Rat caudate synaptosomes. *Science* 27 July: 412.

Lancet. 1981. Editorial: Recurrent urticaria. 2: 235–6.

Lancet. 1985. Editorial: Acid rain and human health. 1: 616–18.

Lessof, M.H. 1983. Food intolerance and allergy — a review. *Quarterly J. Med.* New Series LII (206): 117–19.

Levine, S.A., and Parker, J. 1982. Selenium and human chemical hypersensitivities: preliminary findings. *Int. J. Biosoc. Res.* 3(1): 44–7.

——, 1983. Oxidant/antioxidants and chemical hypersensitivities (part one). *Int. J. Biosoc. Res.* 4(1): 51–4 (part two) 4(2): 102–5.

——, and Reinhardt, J.H. 1983. Biochemical-pathology initiated by free radicals, oxidant chemicals and therapeutic drugs in etiology of chemical hypersensitivity disease. *J. Orthomol. Psychiatry* 12(3): 166–83.

——, and Kidd, P.M. 1985. *Antioxidant adaptation*. Allergy Research Group. San Leandro, California: Biocurrents Division.

Levitan, H. 1979. Food Colours VII Current Issues in Neurotoxicity 185–91 1980. Proceedings of the Fifth FDA Science Symposium: The effects of foods and drugs on the development and function of the nervous system: methods for predicting toxicity, 10–12 October.

Lipton, M.A. 1979. Nemeroff, C.B. and Mailman, R.B. Hyperkinesis and food additives. In *Nutrition and the Brain* 4, Ed. R.J. Wurtman and J.J. Wurtman, 1–27. New York: Raven Press.

Lloyd, A.G., and Drake, J.J.P. 1975. Problems posed by essential food preservatives. *Br. Med. Bull.* 31(3): 214–18.

McGovern, J.J. 1982. Apparent immunotoxic response to phenolic compounds. *Food and Chem. Toxicol.* 20(4): 491.

——, Gardener, R.W., Rapp, D.J., and Painter, K. 1982. Natural foodborne aromatics induce behavioural disturbances in children with hyperkinesis. *Int. J. Biosoc. Dis.* 3: December.

McGraw, M., Bishop, N., O'Hara, M. *et al.* 1986. Aluminium content of milk formulae and intravenous fluids used in infants. *Lancet* 1: 157.

Mailman, R.B., Ferris, R.M., Tang, F.L.M. 1980, Erythrosine (Red No. 3) and its nonspecific biochemical actions: what relation to behaviour changes? *Science* 1 February: 535–7.

Manber, M. 1976. The medical effects of coffee. *Medical World News* 26 January: 63–73.

Marlowe, M., Moon, C., Errera, J. *et al.* 1983. Hair mineral content as a predictor of mental retardation. *J. Orthomol. Psychiatry* 12(1): 26–33.

——, Errera, J. Stellern, J. *et al.* 1983. Lead and mercury levels in emotionally disturbed children *J. Orthomol. Psychiatry.* 12(4): 260–7.

Mason, J., and Singer, P. *Animal Factories.* New York: Crown Publishers.

Mau, G. 1976. Smoking and the fetus. *Lancet* 1: 972.

Michaëlsson, G., and Juhlin, L. 1973. Urticaria induced by preservatives and dye additives in food and drugs. *British Journal of Dermatology* 88: 525–32.

Moore-Robinson, M., and Warin, R.P. 1967. Effect of salicylates in urticaria. *Brit. Med. J.* 4: 262–4.

National Health and Medical Research Council. 1984. Format for the application for the use of a food additive approved by council at the ninety-first session June 1981 through to ninety-eighth session, 1 October, 1984. Canberra: Commonwealth Department of Health.

New Scientist. 1980. Editorial: Court calls for fewer toxins in food. 6: 4 April.

Nutrition Reviews. 1982. Possible vitamin B6 deficiency uncovered in persons with the 'Chinese Restaurant Syndrome'. 40(1): 15–16.

O'Shea, J.A., Porter, S.F. 1981. Double blind study of children with hyperkinetic syndrome treated with multiallergen extracts sublingually. *J. Learning Disabilities* 14(4): 189–91.

Pollak, J.K., Short, K.T., and Verkerk, R.H.J. 1985. A critical analysis of five organochlorine pesticides and implications for their use in NSW. Sydney, Australia: The Toxic and Hazardous

Chemicals Committee of the Total Environment Centre.

Reinland, B. 1983. The Feingold diet: an assessment of the Reviews by Mattes, by Kavale and Forness and others. *J. Learning Disabilities* 16(6): 331–33.

Rice, S.L., Eiten Miller, R.R., and Koehler, P.E. 1976. Biologically active amines in food: a review. *J. Milk Food Technol.* 39(5): 353–8.

Richardson, K.C. 1984. The use of food additives in Australia. *CSIRO Food Res. Quarterly* 44(4): 89–94.

Rippere, V. 1984. Some varieties of food intolerance in psychiatric patients: an overview. *Nutrition and Health* 3(3): 130–1.

Royal College of Physicians, London. 1984. Pharmacological Reactions Associated with Foods. *Journal* 18(2): 110–11.

Sahabat Alam Malaysia (Friends of the Earth). 1981. Pesticide problems in a developing country — a case study of Malaysia. Penang. Malaysia.

Science. 1976. Editorial: Drug resistance growing worse. 194(4272): 1396.

Science. 1976. Editorial: FDA to limit drugs in animal feeds. 196(4289): 510.

Selinger, B. 1981. *Chemistry in the market place.* Canberra: Australian National University Press.

Sohler, A., Pfeiffer C.C., Papaioannou, R. 1981. Blood aluminium levels in a psychiatric outpatient population. High aluminium levels related to memory loss. *J. Orthomol. Psychiatry.* 10(1): 54–60.

Stone, D., Siskind, V., Heinonen, O.P. *et al.* 1976. Aspirin and congenital malformations. *Lancet* 1: 1373–5.

Sutton, P.R.N. 1979. *Fluoridation scientific criticisms and fluoride dangers*: a personal submission to the Committee of Inquiry into the Fluoridation of Victorian Water Supplies, August.

Swanson, J.M., and Kinsbourne, M. 1980. Food dyes impair performance of hyperactive children on a laboratory learning test. *Science* 207 (28 March): 1485–7.

Swain, A., Truswell, A.S., and Loblay, R.H. 1984. Adverse reactions to food. *Food Technology in Australia* 36(10): 467–71.

——, Dutton, S.P., and Truswell, A.S. 1985. Salicylates in foods. *J. of The American Dietetic Association* 85(8): 950–60.

——, Soutter, V., Loblay, R. and Truswell, A.S. 1985. Salicylates, oligoantigenic diets, and behaviour. *Lancet* 2: 41–2.

Total Environment Centre. 1984. Hazardous chemicals in the Australian environment. Proceedings of Conference, August 1983 Sydney, Australia.

Towns, S.J., and Mellis, C.M. 1984. Role of acetyl salicylic acid and sodium metabisulphite in chronic childhood asthma. *Pediatrics* 73(5): 631–7.

United States Dept. of Health and Human Services, Public Health

Service, National Institute of Health. 1984. *Adverse reactions to foods.* NIH Publication 84 July: 2442.

Van Den Bosch, R. 1980. *The pesticide conspiracy.* Dorset, England: Prism Press.

Waldbott, G.L., Burgstahler, A.W., and McKinney, H.L. 1978. Fluoridation: the great dilemma. Lawrence, Kansas: Coronado Press.

Warin, R.P. and Smith, R.J. 1976. Challenge test battery in chronic urticaria. *British Journal of Dermatology.* 94: 401–6.

Weiss, B., Williams, J.H., Abrams, B. *et al.* 1980. Behavioural responses to artificial food colours. *Science* 207 (28 March): 1487–8.

Wraith, D.G. 1984. Specific food allergies. *Chemistry and Industry* 6 February: 95–8.

Wurtman, R.J. and J.J. Wurtman eds. 1983. *Physiological and Behavioural Effects of Food Constituents. Nutrition and the Brain,* volume 6, New York: Raven Press.

Index

2,4,5T (Agent Orange), 137, 146, 151, 188
2,4D, 137, 146, 149, 151, 162
4-hydroxy-benzoic acid, 84
6-hydroxydopamine, 60
abortion rates, 128
accidental poisonings, 147; sprayings, 147
acesulfame potassium, 18
acetoaminophen, 208
acetomethobenzensulphonic acid, 59
acetyl alicylic acid (aspirin), 171
acetylcysteine, 185, 208
acid rain, 109, 110
activated charcoal, 204
acute leukaemia, 147
adrenaline structure, 171
Agent Orange (2,4,5T), 137, 146, 151, 188
aflotoxins, 152
airborne lead, 111
alcohol, 185
aldrin, 137, 138, 143, 151; and Dieldrin residues in food, 135; chemical structure, 136
allergic reactions to water, 207
allergy mediators, 195
Allura Red AC, 13
aluminium, 115, 208; and psychiatric patients, 115; and short-term memory loss, 115; concentration in the brain, 118; containing antacids, 115; in infant milk formulas, 117, 118; in joint tissues, 117, 118; environmental sources of, 116, in neurological disorders, 115
Alzheimers Disease, 116
amalgam corrosion, 109

amalgam fillings, 109; loss of mercury from, 109
amaranth, 12, 84
American white-tailed eagles, 139
amines, 158; biologically active in plant foods, 159
amitrole, 146
amphetamine, 184
amyotrophic lateral sclerosis (ALS), 115
anaerobic exercise, 167
angioedema, 81; challenges for, 82
Animal Factories, 101
Annato, 16
antibiotic dye, Prontosil, 60
antibiotics, 104; in animal feed, 99, 100, 101; residues, 99, 105; resistant bacteria, 100, 102, 105
antibodies, 195
anticaking agents, 3, 19, 22, 27
antidepressant drugs, 157
antidote for fluoride poisoning, 122
antifoaming agents, 3
antimicrobials, 7, 8
antioxidants, 3, 5, 7, 49, 50, 173; chemical structure of, 6; defence system, 173, 174, 179; enzymes, 173, 178; nutrients, 176; nutrition supplements, 205; protective, 174, 209
anxiety, 166; neurosis, 166; states, 166
aplastic leukaemia, 147
apples, chemical to ripen, 154
aromatic compounds, 171
artificial colouring agents, 13, 47, 50, 51
artificial sweetening agents, 18, 90
ascorbic acid, 54, 174, 176, 190, 191,

216

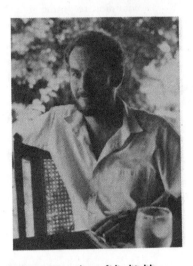

ROBERT BUIST, author of the highly
acclaimed *Food Intolerance*, received his PhD
in Medicinal Chemistry from Macquarie
University in 1974 and completed
postdoctoral studies in the USA in 1976. He
presently is a private consultant specialising
in nutritional medicine and food and
chemical sensitivities. Dr Buist is also the
editor of *International Clinical Nutrition
Review* and lectures extensively to health
professionals and the public, both in
Australia and overseas.